Blood-derived stem cells are used increasingly to treat cancer. This book examines the latest information in this new and rapidly emerging field and assesses its future therapeutic role.

The readable and well-structured text opens with an overview of the concepts behind, and advantages of, blood stem cell transplants. Detailed concepts of their use are later expanded upon and critically reviewed by experts. Among the important issues discussed are hematopoietic recovery, tumor contamination and recent techniques to purify stem cells. Clinical trial data follow including those for leukemia, lymphoma, myeloma and breast cancer. The final chapter evaluates progress in the use of blood stem cells and points to future research and clinical directions.

This is a timely and comprehensive review of the current techniques in blood stem cell transplants and will be welcomed by transplant physicians, oncologists, hematologists and research scientists alike.

GW00546015

BLOOD STEM CELL TRANSPLANTS

BLOOD STEM CELL TRANSPLANTS

Edited by

ROBERT PETER GALE

Associate Professor of Medicine, UCLA School of Medicine, Los Angeles, USA

CHRISTOPHER JUTTNER

Clinical Director, Hanson Centre for Cancer Research, Adelaide, South Australia

PHILIPPE HENON

Head of the Department of Hematology, Director of the Institut de Recherche en Hématologie et Transfusion, Hôpital du Hasenrain, Mulhouse, France

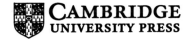
CAMBRIDGE
UNIVERSITY PRESS

CAMBRIDGE UNIVERSITY PRESS

Cambridge, New York, Melbourne, Madrid, Cape Town,
Singapore, São Paulo, Delhi, Tokyo, Mexico City

Cambridge University Press
The Edinburgh Building, Cambridge CB2 8RU, UK

Published in the United States of America by Cambridge University Press, New York

www.cambridge.org
Information on this title: www.cambridge.org/9780521116930

First published 1994
First paperback edition 2011

A catalogue record for this publication is available from the British Library

Library of Congress Cataloguing in Publication data

Blood stem cell transplants / edited by Robert Peter Gale, Christopher Juttner,
Phillippe Henon.
p. cm.
ISBN 0 521 44210 9 (hardback)
1. Hematopoietic stem cells – Transplantation.   2. Cancer –
Treatment.   3. Leukemia – Treatment.   4. Lymphoma – Treatment.
5. Multiple myeloma – Treatment.   6. Breast – Cancer – Teatment.
I. Gale, Robert Peter.   II. Juttner, Christopher.   III. Henon, Philippe.
[DNLM: 1. Hematopoietic Stem Cells – transplantation.   WH 380 B655 1994]
RC271.B59B57   1994
616.99´406 – dc20   93-15870   CIP

ISBN 978-0-521-44210-7 Hardback
ISBN 978-0-521-11693-0 Paperback

Contents

viii   *Contents*

Contributors

Professor K. H. Antman
Harvard Medical School, Boston, MA 02115-6084, USA

Professor J. O. Armitage
University of Nebraska Medical Center, 600 South 42 Street, Omaha, NE 68109-3332, USA

Dr B. Barlogie
University of Arkansas for Medical Sciences, Division of Hematology/ Oncology, 4301 W. Markham, Slot 508, Little Rock, AR 72205-9985, USA

Dr W. Bensinger
Fred Hutchinson Cancer Research Center, 1124 Columbia Street, Seattle, MA 98104-2092, USA

Dr A. C. Eaves
Terry Fox Laboratory, Division of Hematology, British Columbia Cancer Agency, Vancouver General Hospital and University of British Columbia, 601 West 10th Avenue, Vancouver, BC, Canada V5Z 1L3

Dr C. J. Eaves
Medical Genetics, Terry Fox Laboratory, British Columbia Cancer Agency and University of British Columbia, 601 West 10th Avenue, Vancouver, BC, Canada V5Z 1L3

Dr J.-P. Fermand
Laboratoire d'Immunologie et D'Hematologie, Hopital Saint-Louis, 1 Rue C. Vellefaux, 75005 Paris, France

Professor Dr h.c. T. M. Fliedner
Institute of Occupational and Social Medicine, Ulm University, 7900 Ulm, Germany

Professor R. P. Gale
Division Hematology and Oncology, UCLA School of Medicine, Los Angeles, CA 90024-1678, USA

Dr A. M. Gianni
Clinical Therapeutics Institute, Nazionale Tumori, Via Venezian 1, 20153 Milan, Italy

Professor J. M. Goldman
MRC/LRF Leukaemia Unit, Royal Postgraduate Medical School, Ducane Road, London W12 0NN, UK

Dr P. Henon
Institut de Recherche en Hématologie et Transfusion, 87 Avenue d'Altkirch, Hopital du Hasenrain, Pavillon 50, 68100 Mulhouse, France

Dr C. Hoyle
MRC/LRF Leukaemia Unit, Royal Postgraduate Medical School, Ducane Road, London W12 0NN, UK

Dr S. Jagannath
University of Arkansas for Medical Sciences, Division of Hematology/ Oncology, 4301 W. Markham, Slot 508, Little Rock, AK 72205-9985, USA

Dr C. A. Juttner
Leukaemia Research Unit, Hanson Centre for Cancer Research, Institute of Medical and Veterinary Science, Frome Road, Adelaide, SA 5000, Australia

Dr A. Kessinger
Department of Internal Medicine, University of Nebraska Medical Center, Dewey Avenue, Omaha, NE 68198-3330, USA

Dr M. Korbling
Sections of Pheresis and Bone Marrow Transplantation, Department of Hematology/Box 068, The University of Texas, M. D. Anderson Cancer Center, 1515 Holcombe Boulevard, Houston, TX 77030, USA

Dr D. W. Maher
Ludwig Institute for Cancer Research, Melbourne Tumour Biology Branch, Royal Melbourne Hospital, Victoria 3050, Australia

Dr J. Reiffers
Unite de Greffe, Hopital Haut-Leveque, 33604 Pessac, France

Professor J. G. Sharp
Departments of Cell Biology, and Anatomy and Radiology, University of Nebraska Medical Center, 600 South 42 Street, Omaha, NE 68198-6395, USA

Dr W. P. Sheridan
Royal Melbourne Hospital, Victoria 3050, Australia

Dr L. B. To
Leukaemia Research Unit, Hanson Centre for Cancer Research, Institute of Medical and Veterinary Science, Frome Road, Adelaide, SA 5000, Australia

Preface

Transplants of blood-derived stem or progenitor cells are increasingly used to treat cancer. Most of these are autotransplants but there is also recent interest in allogeneic transplants using this approach. There is also recent interest in using blood stem cell transplants in other hematologic, immune and genetic disorders.

Use of blood stem cell transplants in humans is based on considerable experimental data *in vitro* and in animals developed over the past 40 years. Most clinical applications have developed in the past 5 years.

This volume is divided into four sections. First we and our colleagues consider issues involved in blood stem cell transplants and review their history briefly. Part I considers concepts underlying this approach. Part II reviews results of clinical trials in diseases where blood stem cell transplants are most commonly used presently. In Part III the editors have tried to comment critically on the preceding chapters and suggest future research questions.

We hope this volume will be a useful reference for basic and clinical scientists interested in blood stem cell transplants. Practitioners planning to use these transplants and physicians in training should also find it a helpful introduction to this rapidly expanding field.

Robert Peter Gale
Christopher Juttner
Philippe Henon

Los Angeles, Adelaide and Mulhouse

Abbreviations

BCNU	1,3-bis-(2-chloroethyl)-1-nitrosourea
BFU-E	burst-forming unit-erythroid
CCNU	1-2(2-chloroethyl)-3-cyclohexyl-1-nitrosourea
CFU	colony-forming unit
CFU-E	CFU-erythroid
CFU-GEMM	CFU-multilineage progenitor
CFU-GM	CFU-granulocyte/macrophage
CFU-S	CFU-spleen
CRU	competitive repopulating unit
CSF	colony-stimulating factor
DMSO	dimethylsulfoxide
FAB	French–American–British classification of leukemia
FACS	fluorescence activated cell sorter
G-CSF	granulocyte colony-stimulating factor
GM-CSF	granulocyte/macrophage colony-stimulating factor
LTC-IC	long-term culture-initiating cell
LTMC	long-term marrow cultures
MRA	marrow repopulating activity
m^2	body surface area in square metres
Ph	Philadelphia (chromosome)

1

Overview of blood stem cell transplants

R. P. GALE, P. HENON AND C. A. JUTTNER

Introduction

Transplants of blood-derived stem cells are being performed increasingly. Most are autotransplants in persons with cancer. There is also interest in blood stem cell autotransplants in other diseases and as a vehicle for gene therapy. There is even interest in allografts of blood-derived stem cells.

There are no comprehensive reviews of blood stem cell transplants. In this volume we challenged ourselves and our colleagues to discuss recent progress and to suggest future research directions. In this overview we briefly consider important issues in this field. Our objective is to provide the reader with the necessary background to critically evaluate data and views in the chapters that follow. In a final chapter we summarize our conclusions on these issues based on our own data and that of our coauthors. We hope this slightly unorthodox approach will stimulate discussion and debate in this interesting and rapidly emerging field.

Hematopoietic recovery

The two major issues related to hematopoietic recovery after blood stem cell transplants are whether immediate recovery is accelerated and whether there is functional long-term engraftment.

There is little question that granulocyte recovery is more rapid with blood autografts than with bone marrow autografts. This effect is detected only when blood stem cells are collected after mobilization with chemotherapy or hematopoietic growth factors. Accelerated granulocyte recovery is also reported with combinations of mobilized blood and bone marrow cells compared with bone marrow alone.

Accelerated platelet recovery after blood stem cell transplants is less

1

consistent. Why this is so is unknown. Prior bone marrow damage and adverse effects of cryopreservation may be important. Conditions used to collect stem cells may also influence the likelihood of accelerating platelet recovery.

The second issue is whether blood stem cell transplants result in long-term engraftment. Data from animal studies suggest this can occur. Analysis of this question in humans is limited by the lack of an assay for stem cells responsible for long-term engraftment and the absence of data from blood stem cell allografts. It is known that blood stem cell grafts are followed by adequate bone marrow function for more than 5 years posttransplant. Whether this is from the transplanted cells or recovery of endogenous stem cells is unknown. It may be possible to answer this question in the future by using 'genetically marked' stem cells or by allogenic blood stem cell transplants.

Tumor contamination

One argument for using blood rather than bone marrow stem cells is the lower likelihood of the graft containing tumor cells. Is this really so? The answer must be tentative and may differ for different cancers. For example, in autotransplants for leukemia, persisting leukemia cells in the subject are probably the major cause of relapse, and consequently it makes little difference whether blood or bone marrow cells are used for the graft. In lymphoma, in contrast, persons in whom lymphoma cells were detected in the bone marrow graft and who received bone marrow grafts had more relapses than seemingly comparable persons receiving blood cell grafts. It is unknown whether the increased relapse is from the graft per se or whether bone marrow contamination is an adverse risk factor independent of the type of graft.

The major analytic problem in this field is that it is presently impossible to identify tumor cells capable of causing cancer recurrence. For example, the detection of tumor cells in the graft does not mean that they can or do cause relapse. Prospective clinical studies are needed to evaluate their importance. The answer to this question may differ for different cancers.

Hematopoietic growth factors

Hematopoietic growth factors facilitate collecting blood stem cells. Some data suggest that blood stem cells collected after stimulation with different growth factors may have different features. There are no controlled trials showing that posttransplant use of growth factors accelerates granulocyte recovery beyond that reported when chemotherapy or growth factor-mobilized blood stem cells are used alone.

One important issue here is whether reasonably prompt hematopoietic recovery might not be achieved after intensive therapy using hematopoietic growth factors alone without a transplant; the answer is unknown. Most data suggest that growth factors are effective only when sufficient numbers of residual stem cells remain to be stimulated. This is determined by the intensity of therapy used. It is impossible to predict whether treatment with growth factors alone can replace a transplant because the level required to increase cancer cures is not precisely known. The recent trend to use several cycles of less intensive pretransplant chemotherapy rather than one very intensive cycle increases the likelihood that a transplant may not be needed.

Stem cell purification and manipulation

There are several reasons for wanting to obtain pure or enriched hematopoietic stem cells from the blood or bone marrow. One is to decrease the likelihood of transplanting contaminating cancer cells. A second use is to facilitate attempts at *in vitro* growth of these cells or their progeny. So far, there are no convincing data from animals or humans that numbers of stem cells can be increased by *in vitro* culture. Success in this approach might nevertheless have several effects such as reducing the number of leukaphereses needed to collect adequate numbers of blood stem cells for transplantation. Another use might be to provide the greater numbers of stem cells probably needed for allografts (see below). Even if stem cell numbers cannot be increased, growing purified stem cells *in vitro* might provide large numbers of more differentiated progeny that might further accelerate hemotopoietic recovery posttransplantation by providing a type of cell not currently transplanted. A fourth possible use of purified stem cells is as a vehicle to introduce new or modified genes for genetic engineering.

Autotransplants for cancer

Almost all blood stem cell transplants are autotransplants in persons with cancer and therefore a discussion of the validity of principles underlying this approach is central to evaluating the possible efficacy of transplants of blood stem cells.

The use of bone marrow autotransplants in cancer is based on the notion that more intensive therapy is better. Is this really so? Most cancers show a correlation between drug dose and cytotoxicity when tested *in vitro*; however, analyses of data from chemotherapy trials has led to contradictory conclusions in most cancers. Most cancers show a correlation between dose and response, but a correlation between dose and cure is less certain. This controversy exists for several cancers frequently treated by blood stem cell autotransplants, for example acute leukemias, lymphomas, myeloma and breast cancer.

Another important question is whether it is necessary to eradicate all cancer cells to cure cancer. Recent data in acute myelogenous leukemia and follicular lymphomas suggest the malignant clone may persist in persons seemingly cured. If this were so in other cancers, the rationale for dose escalation may be less convincing. In other cancers, such as acute lymphoblastic leukemia, detection of persisting leukemia-related cells seems correlated with relapse. Here, the argument for dose escalation is more compelling, albeit unproven.

There is also difficulty in determining whether results of autotransplants (using blood and or bone marrow cells) are superior to chemotherapy alone. Direct comparison of published data suggest an advantage for autotransplants in some cancers, for example lymphomas and breast cancer. Whether these favorable results of either treatment reflect better therapy or better subjects is unknown. Randomized trials addressing this issue are progressing but more are required.

Allografts of blood stem cells

There are several reasons why blood might be a desirable source of stem cells for allografts, for example, some donors might prefer several leukaphereses to surgery. The more important issue, however, is whether there is reason to think that a blood stem cell transplant would be more likely to engraft or less likely to cause graft-versus-host disease than a bone marrow transplant from the same donor. Most data suggest the opposite. Blood stem cells might accelerate immediate recovery but the important goal here, in contrast to autotransplants, is long-term engraftment. Also, blood stem cell transplants are likely to cause severe graft-versus-host disease because of the higher ratio of T cells to stem cells compared with bone marrow. These T cells can be removed using monoclonal anti-T cell antibodies or by purifying stem cells (see above). This tactic is very likely, however, to increase the risk of graft rejection. Despite these reservations, successful long-term engraftment of blood-derived stem cells is reported in histoincompatible mice and dogs.

Cord blood cell transplants

Recently, successful transplants of stem cells derived from umbilical cord blood were reported in children with Fanconi anemia. This result is not surprising because cord blood cells contain reasonably large numbers of stem cells. There are, unfortunately, no data suggesting that cord blood cells have less immune reactivity than other sources of stem cells. There is no reason consequently, to expect less GVHD after such transplants. This means that the major attraction of cord blood cell transplants is the ability to get cells from very young donors and the possibility of using these cells in persons needing an autotransplant, whose cord blood cells were cryopreserved at birth.

Gene therapy

The major limitation to successful gene therapy today is achieving adequate levels of regulated gene expression in long-lived cells. Purified blood stem cells might help by increasing the likelihood of introducing the desired gene into a stem cell. Apart from technical considerations, however, there is no reason why blood stem cells should be superior to those from the bone marrow; they may be worse as the frequency of very long lived cells is probably less.

Conclusion

In this overview we raise issues underlying the use and analysis of blood stem cell transplants. We hope these serve as a basis for considering the chapters that follow, in which most of these issues are discussed in greater detail. In the final chapter we use data presented here and in the rest of this volume to try to answer some of these questions.

Part I

Concepts

2

History of blood stem cell transplants

M. KORBLING AND T. M. FLIEDNER

Introduction

There are few areas in experimental hematology research that have seen more advances in the past few decades than those concerned with the physiology and pathophysiology of the kinetics, function and regulation of the hematopoietic cell renewal systems, particularly their stem cell populations. In the 1950s, the major tool of hematology was that of cellular morphology supplemented by cytochemical approaches. In the 1960s, the methodological literature was abundant with the characterization of the turnover kinetics of hematopoietic cell systems. By the 1970s, bone marrow transplantation was recognized as a therapeutic approach in the treatment of various malignant lymphohematopoietic disorders and aplastic anemia, and in the 1980s, growth factors and regulation of the hematopoietic cell systems became the dominant interest of research.

Hematopoietic stem cell migration via the blood has been known and appreciated for decades. Maximow (Fig. 2.1) postulated as early as 1909, when he gave a talk 'in der ausserordentlichen Sitzung der Berliner Hämatologischen Gesellschaft' at the famous Charité Hospital, that the lymphocyte acts as a common stem cell and migrates through tissues to seed in appropriate microenvironments. In the 1950s, stem cell migration was demonstrated in radiological studies. The shielding of part of the hematopoietic tissue or part of the blood circulation during lethal total body irradiation results in the subsequent reconstitution of the marrow in the irradiated areas. C.E. Ford, H.S. Micklem, E.P. Cronkite and others, using chromosomal markers, showed that this was the result of migration of pluripotent stem cells from the shielded to the irradiated marrow areas. The basic concept of 'stem cell transplantation' was born.

Stem cell migration is also part of the concept of fetal hematopoietic development. Stem cells appear to migrate to 'ecological niches', an

Der Lymphozyt als gemeinsame Stammzelle
der verschiedenen Blutelemente in der embryonalen
Entwicklung und im postfetalen Leben der Säugetiere.[1]

Von

Prof. Dr. A. Maximow.

[1] Demonstrationsvortrag, gehalten in der ausserordentlichen Sitzung der Berliner Hämatologischen Gesellschaft am 1. Juni 1909.

Folia Haemat (Lpz.) 8, 1909

Fig. 2.1. Maximow postulates in 1909 that lymphocytes act as a common stem cell.

expression created by T.M. Fliedner, such as in the liver and bone marrow, via the vitelline, but even more so, the allantoic circulation. It has been of great interest, in this context, to establish that each site of developing bone marrow experiences a short period of 'hematopoietic aplasia', during which it consists only of a vascularized 'cellular matrix', before it becomes hematopoietic as a result of the immigration and extravasation of hematopoietic stem cells. Thus, if stem cell transfusion in the adult can lead to repopulation of an aplastic marrow, the prenatal development of hematopoiesis would in a certain sense, appear to be repeated.

In the early 1960s, stem cells had been shown to be permanent residents of the peripheral blood, as part of the mononuclear leukocyte population. Joan Goodman and George Hodgson from Oak Ridge National Laboratory (Fig. 2.2) first used the term 'blood stem cell' in a paper published in 1962. They were the first to show definite evidence that circulating stem cells are capable of restoring irradiation-myeloablated hematopoiesis in mice.

Intensive experimental stem cell research started during the same period. Till and McCulloch introduced the 'spleen colony assay', and the research group of E.D. Thomas, at that time still in Cooperstown, NY, investigated the principles of clinical bone marrow transplantation using the dog model. Thomas' group confirmed earlier findings in mice; among the circulating blood leukocytes are indeed cells that have the potential to completely reverse a radiation-induced myeloablation. In the autologous transplant

Evidence for Stem Cells in the Peripheral Blood of Mice

By JOAN WRIGHT GOODMAN AND GEORGE S. HODGSON

Blood 19, 1962

Fig. 2.2. Goodman and Hodgson first introduce the term 'blood stem cell' into the literature in 1962.

The Recovery of Lethally Irradiated Dogs Given Infusions of Autologous Leukocytes Preserved at –80 C.

By JOHN A. CAVINS, STUART C. SCHEER, E. DONNALL THOMAS AND JOSEPH W. FERREBEE

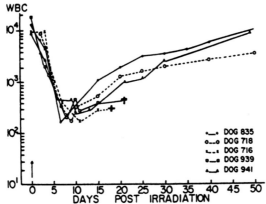

Fig. 1.—Peripheral white blood cell counts of dogs exposed to 1200 r of Co⁶⁰ radiation and given an infusion of a sample of autologous white cells that had been stored at −80 C. in 10 per cent dimethylsulfoxide.

Blood 23, 1964

Fig. 2.3. Cavins and colleagues successfully transplant cryopreserved blood stem cells into irradiated dogs.

situation, Cavins and colleagues (Fig. 2.3) were the first to successfully transplant cryopreserved blood stem cells into dogs, and Storb and Epstein (Fig. 2.4) performed similar studies in the allogeneic transplant situation by utilizing, among others, the elegant cross-circulation experiments.

Fliedner and his group, first at the Brookhaven National Laboratory during 1958, then in Freiburg, West Germany, in 1964, described mononuclear cells in human circulating blood that were capable of dividing. One has to understand that at that time it was believed that immature cells did not circulate in human blood and, if present, might indicate leukemic malignancy. The stem cells responsible for hematopoietic reconstitution are quiescent under steady state conditions but when they are taken off the G_0 phase they enter the cell cycle and replicate and differentiate.

Stem cells are in dynamic equilibrium between blood and extravascular sites, as was demonstrated by extensive leukapheresis. In dog experiments, performed in Ulm in 1978, more than 100 times the number of colony-

M. Korbling and T. M. Fliedner

**Marrow Engraftment by Allogeneic Leukocytes in
Lethally Irradiated Dogs**

By R. Storb, R. B. Epstein, H. Ragde, J. Bryant and E. D. Thomas

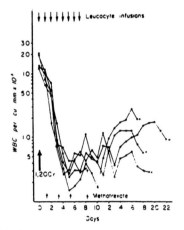

Fig. 1.—White blood cells per cu. mm. in dogs given 1200 r of whole-bod
irradiation, allogeneic leukocytes and methotrexate.

Blood 30, 1967

Demonstration of Hemopoietic Stem Cells in the Peripheral Blood of Baboons by Cross Circulation

By Rainer Storb, Theodore C. Graham, Robert B. Epstein, George E. Sale,
and E. Donnall Thomas

Blood 50, 1977

Fig. 2.4. Storb and Epstein carry out their elegant cross-circulation experiments to
prove the reconstitutive potential of the blood stem cell.

forming units granulocyte/macrophage (CFU-GM) present in the total
blood volume at a given time was removed within 24 hours without
exhausting the blood or bone marrow CFU-GM pools. Thus one more
'brick' in the concept of blood stem cell transplants was added.

Preclinical experiments became more sophisticated: blood stem cell
purification yielded a ratio of 1 CFU-GM of 13 blood mononuclear cells,
and allogeneic transplantation of those purified blood stem cell suspensions
resulted in complete hematopoietic engraftment without GVHD (Fig. 2.5).
Finally, cytogenetic studies after allogeneic blood stem cell transplants left
no doubt that blood-derived hematopoietic stem cells sustain hematopoietic

Albumin Density Gradient Purification of Canine Hemopoietic Blood Stem Cells (HBSC): Long-Term Allogeneic Engraftment Without GVH-Reaction

MARTIN KÖRBLING*, THEODOR M. FLIEDNER, WENCESLAO CALVO,
WILLIAM M. ROSS, WILHELM NOTHDURFT & IRMHILD STEINBACH
(with the assistance of INGE FACHE & ESTHER RÜBER)

Department of Clinical Physiology, University of Ulm, Federal Republic of Germany

Experimental Hematology 7, 1979

Cytogenetic Studies in Dogs after Total Body Irradiation and Allogeneic Transfusion with Cryopreserved Blood Mononuclear Cells: Observations in Long-Term Chimeras

*Felix Carbonell, Wenceslao Calvo, Theodor M. Fliedner,
Elisabeth Kratt, Heinrich Gerhartz, Martin Körbling,
Wilhelm Nothdurft, William M. Ross*

Department of Clinical Physiology and Occupational Medicine.
University of Ulm. Oberer Eselsberg. Ulm. West Germany

Intern J Cell Cloning 2: 81-88, 1984

Fig. 2.5. In allogeneic transplantation experiments, Fliedner's group demonstrates the long-term hematopoietic engraftment capability of the blood stem cell. Reproduced with the permission of AlphaMed press and The Journal of the International Society for Experimental Hematology.

reconstitution after transplantation for more than 10 years (Fig. 2.5). The conclusion was that under transplant conditions the blood-derived stem cell is qualitatively equivalent to the marrow-derived stem cell.

There was, however, concern about the proliferative potential of circulating stem cells. Micklem and colleagues (Fig. 2.6) from Edinburgh University, doubted a sufficient self-renewal capacity of the blood stem cell. It seemed to them 'reasonable to speculate that the CFUs normally found in blood are victims of clonal senescence, and have been expelled as waste products from the bone marrow'.

Together with the development of the IBM blood cell separator, Kenneth McCredie, Evan Hersh and Emil Freireich (Fig. 2.7) were the first to perform clinical trials on the separation and collection of blood stem cells at the M.D. Anderson Cancer Center in Houston. Those data were

M. Korbling and T. M. Fliedner

Limited potential of circulating haemopoietic stem cells

Nature, Vol.256, 1975   H. S. MICKLEM
N. ANDERSON
ELIZABETH ROSS

*Department of Zoology,
University of Edinburgh,
West Mains Road,
Edinburgh EH9 3JT, UK*

Fig. 2.6. Micklem and colleagues express concern about the proliferative potential of circulating stem cells, and speculate on their being waste products. Reprinted with permission from *Nature*, **256**, 1975, Macmillan Magazines Limited.

Cells Capable of Colony Formation in the Peripheral Blood of Man

Number of colonies per plate in stimulated cultures of peripheral blood and leukapheresis leukocytes collected and cultured simultaneously at 2×10^6 nucleated cells per plate for 14 days.

Source of inoculum	No. of subjects	Colonies				Positive colonies (%)
		Mean No.	Median No.	Mean No. in positive cultures	Median No. in positive cultures	
Peripheral blood	29	18	9	30	28	58
Leukapheresis leukocytes	29	23	11	34	21	65

KENNETH B. MCCREDIE
EVAN M. HERSH
EMIL J FREIREICH

*Department of Developmental
Therapeutics, University of Texas,
M. D. Anderson Hospital and Tumor
Institute, Houston 77025*

Science 171, 1971

Collection of Large Quantities of Granulocyte/Macrophage Progenitor Cells (CFUc) in Man by Means of Continuous-Flow Leukapheresis

MARTIN KÖRBLING,[1] THEODOR M. FLIEDNER[1] & HORST PFLIEGER[2]

[1] *Department of Clinical Physiology and* [2] *Department of Internal Medicine,
Division of Haematology, University of Ulm, Ulm, West Germany*

Scand J Haematol 24: 22-28, 1980

Fig. 2.7. First clinical trials on the separation and collection of blood stem cells. Scand. J. Haematol., **24**: 22–28, reproduced with the permission of the authors and © 1980 Munksgaard International Publishers Ltd., Copenhagen, Denmark; and © 1971 by AAAS and McCredie *et al.*, *Science*, **171**: 293–4.

Early Bone Marrow Recovery After Chemotherapy
Following The Transfusion Of
Peripheral Blood Leukocytes In Identical Twins

B.McCredie, E.J Freireich, E.M.Hersh, J.E.Curtis, H.Kaizer

M.D.Anderson Hospital and Tumor Institute,
Houston, Texas

Leukapheresis with the IBM Blood Cell Separator was performed on 3 identical twin donors for 4-5 consecutive days and the leukocytes were transfused into their identical siblings who had received chemotherapy for disseminated malignancies. A total dose of approximately $1x10^{11}$ leukocytes were transfused into each recipient.

Results showed that despite an increase in the dose of chemotherapy the periods of leukopenia and the period of myelosuppression was shortened in each transfused subject.

Serial bone marrows performed on one patient showed that bone marrow cellularity was 10% or less for greater than 21 days after chemotherapy without leukocyte transfusions. A subsequent course of chemotherapy with an increase in dose (33%), followed immediately with 4 days of leukocyte transfusions showed a marrow cellularity of 30% at 15 days and 35% at 18 days.

The transfusion of peripheral blood leukocytes induced early marrow recovery from chemotherapy. The data suggests that stem cells for marrow repopulation exist in the peripheral blood of man.

Proc Am Assoc Cancer Res 11, 1970 (abstr.)

Fig. 2.8. McCredie and Freireich report a clinical transplant experiment in identical twins using peripheral blood leukocytes.

published in *Science* in 1971 and it was almost 10 years before the studies were continued by Fliedner's group at Ulm University (Fig. 2.7). McCredie and Freireich were also the first to perform the clinical leukocyte or blood stem cell transplant experiment in identical twins (Fig. 2.8).

Two attempts were performed almost a decade later to produce engraftment with syngeneic blood stem cells; one was unsuccessful and the other partly successful. Abrams and colleagues administered large numbers of syngeneic blood stem cells to a patient with Ewing's sarcoma who had received intensive consolidation therapy. Lymphocyte recovery was accelerated but there was no change in the speed of recovery of granulocytes or platelets (Fig. 2.9). Hershko and colleagues also failed to cure marrow aplasia in a patient with paroxysmal nocturnal hemoglobinuria by transfusion of white cells from an identical twin. A bone marrow graft from the same donor produced prompt recovery (Fig. 2.9). Failure of engraftment in the first case probably was a result of insufficient numbers of

CURE OF APLASTIC ANÆMIA IN PAROXYSMAL NOCTURNAL HÆMOGLOBINURIA BY MARROW TRANSFUSION FROM IDENTICAL TWIN: FAILURE OF PERIPHERAL-LEUCOCYTE TRANSFUSION TO CORRECT MARROW APLASIA

C. HERSHKO   R. P. GALE
W. G. Ho   M. J. CLINE

*Division of Hematology-Oncology, Department of Medicine,
University of California School of Medicine, Los Angeles,
California 90024, U.S.A.*

The Lancet, May 5, 1979

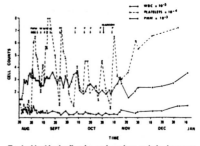

Total white-blood-cell, polymorphonuclear, and platelet counts before and after bone-marrow transfusion.
Arrows indicate platelet (P) and white-blood-cell (W) transfusions.

Result of Attempted Hematopoietic Reconstitution Using Isologous, Peripheral Blood Mononuclear Cells: A Case Report

By R. A. Abrams, D. Glaubiger, F. R. Appelbaum, and A. B. Deisseroth

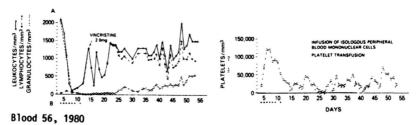

Blood 56, 1980

Fig. 2.9. Two clinical attempts to produce complete hematopoietic engraftment with syngeneic blood stem cells. Reproduced with permission of *The Lancet*.

progenitor cells being transfused. In the second, a higher cell dose was given but the infusions were given intermittently over a 14-day period, a schedule which is thought not to favor engraftment. Those data were very discouraging.

The question was: was stem cell mobilization into the circulating blood needed to guarantee successful engraftment? Carol Richman and colleagues (Fig. 2.10) were the first to use a total stem cell number by multiple apheresis, equivalent to a bone marrow autograft. This regimen is still 15 years later the basic clinical approach to transiently increase blood stem cell concentration.

With the autologous blood stem cell transplant program at Hammersmith Hospital in London, lead by John Goldman (Fig. 2.11), this new technology was rapidly accepted. The clinical transplant data on chronic myelogenous leukemia (CML) patients were somewhat disappointing but autologous blood stem cell transplantation from now on was increasingly considered to be the new therapeutic transplant approach. John Goldman deserves all credit for moving this field a great step ahead.

Increase in Circulating Stem Cells Following Chemotherapy in Man

By Carol M. Richman, Roy S. Weiner, and Ronald A. Yankee

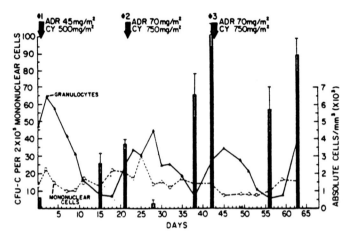

Fig. 1. Serial absolute granulocyte counts (▲——▲), mononuclear cell (lymphocytes + monocytes) counts (⋮-----⋮), and mean peripheral blood CFU-C values (■) following three successive courses of adriamycin (ADR) and cyclophosphamide (CY) for patient No. 1. The dose of drug and day of administration are shown by the arrows. Vertical bars represent SEM.

Blood 47, 1976

Fig. 2.10. Richman and colleagues successfully mobilize stem cells into the circulating blood.

Buffy Coat Autografts for Patients with Chronic Granulocytic Leukaemia in Transformation

J.M. Goldman, D. Catovsky, A.W.G. Goolden, S.A. Johnson, and D.A.G. Galton

MRC Leukaemia Unit and the Department of Radiotherapy,
Royal Postgraduate Medical School, Hammersmith Hospital, Ducane Road,
London W12 OHS, Great Britain

Blut 42, 1981

Fig. 2.11. Goldman at Hammersmith Hospital, London, initiates an autologous blood stem cell transplant programme for chronic myelogenous leukemia as a new therapeutic approach.

At the same time, the leukemia group headed by Phil Burke at the Johns Hopkins Hospital tried to use 'normal' hematopoietic precursor cells for engraftment, collected in a so-called 'true remission' phase of CML without evidence of the Ph^1 chromosome (Fig. 2.12). Although the clinical experiment was not conclusive, they were able to describe the characteristic

M. Korbling and T. M. Fliedner

Successful Engraftment of Blood Derived Normal Hemopoietic Stem Cells in Chronic Myelogenous Leukemia

Martin Körbling, Philip Burke, Hayden Braine, Gerald Elfenbein, George Santos & Herbert Kaizer

The Johns Hopkins Oncology Center, 600 N. Wolfe Street, Baltimore, MD 21205, USA

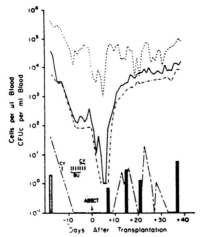

Figure 1. Platelet (- - - - -), WBC (——), PMN (—·—·—·) and CFU$_c$/ml of peripheral blood (— · — · —) and in bone marrow (per 2×10^6 mononuclear marrow cells, stippled bars) before and after autologous blood stem cell transplantation (ABSCT).

Experimental Hematology 9, 1981

Fig. 2.12. The Johns Hopkins' leukemia and bone marrow transplant group first describes the successful autologous transplantation of normal, Philadelphia-negative blood stem cells leading to fast hematopoietic reconstitution. Reproduced with the permission of The Journal of the International Society for Experimental Hematology.

fast reconstitution of white blood cells after myeloablative treatment and autologous blood stem cell transplants.

Since 1985–86, we have known for certain about the clinical hematopoietic reconstitution capability of blood-derived stem cells. Four groups (Fig. 2.13) in different parts of the world, almost simultaneously, carried out clinical experiments showing that normal blood stem cells, transfused as an autograft, function and give permanent rise to all cell lines. These

History

Circulating autologous stem cells collected in
very early remission from acute non-lymphoblastic
leukaemia produce prompt but incomplete
haemopoietic reconstitution after high dose
melphalan or supralethal chemoradiotherapy

C. A. JUTTNER, L. B. TO, D. N. HAYLOCK, A. BRANFORD AND R. J. KIMBER
Leukaemia Research Unit, Division of Haematology, Institute of Medical and Veterinary Science, Adelaide, and Clinical Haematology Unit, Royal Adelaide Hospital, Adelaide, South Australia

British Journal of Haematology 61, 1985

Autologous Transplantation of Blood-Derived Hemopoietic Stem Cells After
Myeloablative Therapy in a Patient With Burkitt's Lymphoma

By Martin Körbling, Bernd Dörken, Anthony D. Ho, Antonio Pezzutto, Werner Hunstein, and Theodor M. Fliedner

Blood 67, 1986

Successful Autologous Transplantation with Peripheral Blood Hemopoietic Cells in a Patient with Acute Leukemia

Josy Reiffers, Philippe Bernard, Bernard David, Gérard Vezon, Anne Sarrat, Gérald Marit,
Jacques Moulinier, and Antoine Broustet
Service des Maladies du Sang and the Laboratoire d'Hémobiologie, Bordeaux, Hôpital Haut Lévêque, Pessac; and Centre de Transfusion Sanguine, Bordeaux, France

Experimental Hematology 14, 1986

Reconstitution of Human Hematopoietic Function with Autologous Cryopreserved Circulating Stem Cells

Anne Kessinger,[1] James O. Armitage,[1] James D. Landmark,[2,3] and Dennis D. Weisenburger[3]
Departments of [1]Internal Medicine and [3]Pathology and Laboratory Medicine, University of Nebraska Medical Center; and [2]American Red Cross Blood Services, Midwest Region, Omaha, Nebraska, USA

Experimental Hematology 14, 1986

Fig. 2.13. Simultaneous demonstration by four groups that blood stem cells reconstitute hematopoietic function after myeloablative treatment. Reproduced with the permission of The Journal of the International Society for Experimental Hematology.

investigators included Chris Juttner's group in Adelaide, South Australia, Josy Reiffers' group in Bordeaux, France, Martin Körbling's group in Heidelberg, Germany, and Anne Kessinger's group in Omaha, Nebraska, USA. From that time, literature on the clinical use of blood stem cells expanded, differentiated and maturated.

The historical perspectives mentioned are not complete by far. We wanted to show the enormous scientific achievement and the clinical encouragement which has made our current level of knowledge possible. Today, the autologous blood stem cell transplant field is still developing and blood stem cells are being highly purified and even used as an almost indefinitely self-renewing target population for genetic engineering.

3

ˌu progenitor cells in the blood
C.J. EAVES AND A.C. EAVES

Introduction

The production of blood cells is a complex multistep process involving changes that span many cell generations. During the latter stages of this process, there is normally a partially realized exponential expansion of morphologically recognizable cells of increasing maturity derived from lineage-restricted precursors. These events have been well defined by time lapse photography *in vitro* (e.g. Cormack, 1976) and autoradiographic analysis of cells produced *in vivo* (reviewed by Jandl, 1987). Prior to the acquisition of morphological evidence of differentiation along a particular lineage, however, there are many additional earlier stages of hematopoietic cell development. Terminally differentiating hematopoietic cells are normally confined to the extravascular spaces in the bone marrow but many of the earlier types of hematopoietic cells, like the mature blood cells they ultimately produce, are found in the circulation albeit at low levels (Sutherland *et al.*, 1991a). This chapter reviews methodologies currently available for quantifying and characterizing different types of primitive hematopoietic cells and their relevance to peripheral blood cell transplants.

What is a hematopoietic stem cell?

Most of our concepts about hematopoietic stem cells derive from experiments with bone marrow transplants in lethally irradiated mice. Early recognition that radiation inactivation of dividing blood cell precursors was the most important factor limiting survival after low doses of whole body irradiation led to attempts to quantify the hematopoietic cells which, on transplantation, were responsible for myeloprotection (McCulloch & Till, 1960). It was during the course of these studies that the

Toronto group made their seminal discovery and characterization of a population of pluripotent cells in normal mouse bone marrow that could generate macroscopically visible multilineage colonies of cells in the spleens of histocompatible irradiated recipients (Till & McCulloch, 1961). These spleen colonies were also found to contain new pluripotent cells capable of generating multilineage colonies in the spleens of secondary recipients (Siminovitch *et al.*, 1963). Thus, the existence in adult marrow of a pluripotent hematopoietic cell with the ability to maintain its pluripotential status through several divisions was firmly established. The studies of the Toronto group were additionally important because they introduced the concept of devising quantitative methods to enumerate primitive hematopoietic cells based on the use of endpoints that measure their developmental potential. In parallel was their timely introduction of operational terminology for cells defined by functional assays (e.g. CFU-S for colony-forming unit-spleen).

During the three decades that have elapsed since the discovery of CFU-S, the creation of additional functional assays for primitive hematopoietic cells has expanded to yield a profusion of methodologies and a confusion of terminologies. The exact relationships between the cells detected by these different assays is not yet known because it has rarely been possible to obtain homogeneous populations where even one cell type reads out at 100% efficiency. The picture has also been made more difficult to analyze by a growing body of evidence that the same response of a given precursor may be achieved by its interaction with different growth factors (and/or inhibitors) thus limiting the potential for defining specific cell types on the basis of their factor responsiveness (see e.g. Dexter & Spooncer, 1987; Axelrad, 1990; Sutherland *et al.*, 1991b; Leary *et al.*, 1992). In spite of the recognition of more than 20 such factors active on hematopoietic cell targets, it is likely that additional factors of as yet unknown molecular identity exist. Some of these may already be important components of existing assays (Sutherland *et al.*, 1993).

Definitions of hematopoietic stem cells vary according to the context in which they are to be considered. The most stringent definitions are usually based on the assumption that all hematopoietic cell differentiation steps are irreversible and hence, biologically, the ultimate hematopoietic stem cell population is one whose members will regenerate and sustain long-term production of all other cells in the system. Analysis of the reconstituted hematopoietic tissues of recipients of hematopoietic cells bearing genetic markers has revealed the existence in both small and large animals, including humans, of normal hematopoietic cells that are individually capable of producing many or even most of the blood cells required for many months (Wu *et al.*, 1968; Dick *et al.*, 1985; Lemischka *et al.*, 1986; Turhan *et al.*, 1989; Abkowitz *et al.*, 1990; Keller & Snodgrass, *et al.*, 1990). Such cells would be of prime importance for clinical applications requiring permanent reconstitution of the hematopoietic system with donor-derived cells. On the other hand, there is now growing evidence that such cells may be developmentally unable to generate mature progeny within the time frame required for myeloprotection from lethal doses of chemotherapy or radiation (Ploemacher & Brons, 1988; Jones *et al.*, 1989, 1990). Consequently, in many clinical settings the number of the most primitive hematopoietic cells in a transplant may be less important than the number of intermediate progenitor cell types with only transient repopulating potential but capable of more rapid production of mature cells.

Quantitative assays for primitive hematopoietic cells

At present, although totipotent hematopoietic cells with long-term reconstituting ability are known to exist in human bone marrow (Turhan *et al.*, 1989; Baum *et al.*, 1992), there is no established assay for their quantification, nor is there any clear value in any existing progenitor assay for independently predicting either neutrophil or platelet recovery. Both are important issues and are currently the subject of active investigation.

Two complementary approaches are being used to develop assays for the most primitive human hematopoietic cells that will not only allow their numbers to be measured in various test populations but will also embody sufficient specificity to exclude cells with more restricted, short-term repopulating ability. One approach is to develop an appropriate *in vivo* assay for long-term murine repopulating cells, then to establish an *in vitro* assay that detects this same cell type and finally to demonstrate that the *in vitro* assay can be adapted to detect analogous primitive hematopoietic cells of human origin. Considerable controversy remains concerning the position of CFU-S in the murine hematopoietic cell hierarchy but, it is now clear that many, and perhaps even most, CFU-S are not capable of long-term repopulation (Ploemacher & Brons, 1988; Jones *et al.*, 1990; Smith *et al.*, 1991). Accordingly, other assays focused on longer term endpoints of hematopoietic recovery have had to be developed. Considerable progress along these lines has been made with the development of the CRU (competitive repopulating unit) assay (Szilvassy *et al.*, 1990). CRU and LTC-IC (long-term culture-initiating cells) (Ploemacher *et al.*, 1989; Sutherland *et al.*, 1990) have similar properties that are not shared by most

CFU-S (Ploemacher & Brons, 1989; Ploemacher *et al.*, 1991; Eaves *et al.*, 1992). The CRU assay is an *in vivo* limiting dilution assay which quantifies cells that are individually capable of regenerating at least 5% of the entire hematopoietic system, including both myeloid and lymphoid compartments (Szilvassy *et al.*, 1989a, 1990) and then maintaining the production of these cells for at least 6 months (Fraser *et al.*, 1992). The specificity of the CRU assay for cells with these developmental properties is provided by the requirement (inherent in the design of the assay) that CRU-derived progeny be produced in recipients that have been simultaneously transplanted with other cells that are themselves myeloprotective (e.g. contain ∼30 CFU-S) but have reduced long-term repopulating potential (Szilvassy *et al.*, 1989b, 1990). CFU-S production in the marrow after 2 weeks (referred to as marrow repopulating activity, MRA) may represent an endpoint for a cell that is closely related to CRU (Ploemacher & Brons, 1989). A more complete definition of the developmental properties of MRA cells has not been obtained however, no doubt in part because the MRA assay has the significant disadvantage that only relative changes in MRA can be measured.

LTC-IC are hematopoietic cells that give rise to mature cells after an interval of many weeks in the long-term marrow culture system (Sutherland *et al.*, 1990; Eaves *et al.*, 1991a). As *in vivo*, the mature cells (granulocytes and macrophages) produced in this culture system are in a state of constant turnover (Slovick *et al.*, 1984; Cashman *et al.*, 1985) so that continued maintenance of their numbers depends on the proliferation and differentiation of cells ultimately at a very primitive level of hematopoietic cell development (Sutherland *et al.*, 1989). To ensure that the output of mature cells is strictly a function of the input precursor population, regardless of the number or concentration of such cells in the population to be assayed, each LTC-IC assay culture is provided with a preformed layer of supportive fibroblasts. These may be obtained by subculturing cells from the adherent layer of LTC established 2–6 weeks previously from normal allogeneic human marrow or, alternatively, various murine fibroblast cell lines can be used (Sutherland *et al.*, 1991b). Absolute LTC-IC frequencies can then be determined by limiting dilution analysis using any one of several endpoints to measure LTC-IC function; e.g. the total number of clonogenic myeloid progenitors present after 5 or 8 weeks (Sutherland *et al.*, 1990) (or in the mouse the presence after 4–6 weeks of visible areas of granulopoiesis referred to as cobblestone areas (Ploemacher *et al.*, 1989)). The interval of time allowed to elapse before the differentiated progeny of LTC-IC are assessed is a crucial parameter. Measurement of clonogenic cell numbers at earlier times (i.e. less than 5 weeks after initiation of human LTC-IC assay

Table 3.1. *Properties of LTC-initiating cells*

Frequencies in normal adult tissue	1/20 000 bone marrow cells 3 per ml of blood
Phenotype (differences from clonogenic cells)	Small (low FLS, like lymphocytes) Light ($<1.068\,g/mm^3$) $CD34^{++}$ HLA-DR$\pm$ $CD45RO^+$ $CD71\pm$ Rhodamine-123 dull 4HC-insensitive Slowly cycling
Proliferative potential in LTC (no. of clonogenic cells at 5 weeks)	Mean $=4$ Range $= 1$–30
Differentiation potential in LTC	$\sim 20\%$ are pluripotent
Self-maintenance in LTC	100% after 10 days 25% after 4–5 weeks

LTC, long-term culture; FLS, fluorescence.

cultures) does not allow adequate discrimination between residual input clonogenic cells, clonogenic cells derived from intermediate-type progenitors, and progenitors with features associated more exclusively with long-term repopulating cells when these various types of cells are all represented in the initial test population at frequencies typical of normal hematopoietic tissue (Sutherland *et al.*, 1989; Ploemacher *et al.*, 1989, 1991). The existence of a linear relationship between LTC-IC input and the number of clonogenic cells present 5 weeks later, plus the knowledge that the average clonogenic cell output of individual LTC-IC appears to be invariant (on average, one human LTC-IC generates approximately four clonogenic cells detectable 5 weeks after initiation of the LTC-IC assay culture), allows absolute LTC-IC numbers to be simply calculated from total clonogenic progenitor output values (in assays of human cells, by dividing by 4) (Sutherland *et al.*, 1990; Udomsakdi *et al.*, 1992b).

Table 3.1 shows the properties of human LTC-IC emphasizing features that distinguish them from the majority of clonogenic cells in normal adult marrow. It is important to note that at least some murine CRU proliferate and amplify their numbers significantly in the LTC system (Fraser *et al.*, 1992), although overall the CRU population appears to decline with kinetics very similar to those described for human LTC-IC (Eaves *et al.*, 1991b; Udomsakdi *et al.*, 1992b). These latter findings provide strong support for the concept that LTC-IC and CRU are closely related, if not identical, populations.

An alternative approach to the development of a quantitative assay for human long-term repopulating hematopoietic cells has been to develop strategies for supporting/eliciting this function in suitably prepared xenogeneic hosts (Dick, 1991; Srour *et al.*, 1992). Recently much attention has been focused on the use of severely immunocompromized mice as potential assay recipients of human cells. Some advances using this approach have been made and it is now possible to detect the progeny of human progenitors transplanted into mice several months previously if the latter are provided either with a suitable tissue source of supportive human factors and/or with repeated injections of human species-specific growth factors (Namikawa *et al.*, 1990; Kyoizumi *et al.*, 1992; Lapidot *et al.*, 1992). The frequency and efficiency of human hematopoiesis obtained thus far has not yet allowed this approach to form the basis of a reliable assay for quantifying hematopoietic repopulating cells of human origin.

Intermediate between CRU/LTC-IC and the majority of clonogenic cells detectable by standard assays for granulopoietic (CFU-GM), erythropoietic (BFU-E) and multilineage progenitors (CFU-GEMM) are cells referred to as HPP-CFC (high proliferative potential colony-forming cells, including those stimulated by fibroblasts (Dowding & Gordon, 1992), as well as certain growth factors or combinations of growth factors) (McNiece *et al.*, 1989; Leary *et al.*, 1992) and ΔCFC (net increase in CFC detected after 1 week in culture (Moore, 1991). All of these latter types of progenitors are characterized by a large proliferative capacity demonstrable either in terms of the size of the primary colony generated or by an ability to give rise to daughter clonogenic cells within a 1–2-week time frame of primary colony growth, which are then detected by replating into secondary colony assays.

Primitive hematopoietic cells in the circulation

The presence of primitive hematopoietic cells in adult peripheral blood has been appreciated for several decades. Initial experiments demonstrated the myeloprotective activity of transplanted peripheral blood cells and showed that restoration of hematopoiesis was from the injected blood cells (Brecher & Cronkite, 1951; Goodman & Hodgson, 1962; Cavins *et al.*, 1964; Epstein *et al.*, 1966; Storb *et al.*, 1977; Abrams *et al.*, 1980). Subsequent studies revealed the presence of specific progenitor populations in the circulation detectable by colony assays. Table 3.2 shows normal levels of several of these intermediate progenitor types as determined by

Table 3.2. *Clonogenic progenitor numbers in normal blood and bone marrow*

Progenitor	Blood Mean per ml (± 2 s.d.)	Bone marrow Mean per 2×10^5 nucleated cells (± 2 s.d.)
CFU-E	19 (1–274)	67 (15–305)
BFU-E	106 (17–669)	56 (15–208)
CFU-GM	39 (4–377)	62 (19–201)
CFU-GEMM	3 (0.1–85)	1 (0.04–8)

Based on individual assessments of up to 126 blood samples and 87 bone marrow samples from different normal donors. Assay reagents were optimized and standardized to give the same maximal plating efficiency for light density blood cells and red cell-depleted, but otherwise unseparated, normal human marrow aspirate samples.
CFU-E, colony-forming unit-erythroid; BFU-E, burst-forming unit-erythroid; GEMM, multi-lineage progenitor; GM, granulocyte/macrophage; s.d., standard deviation.
Sources: Sutherland *et al.* (1991a); Udomsakdi *et al.* (1992c).

analysis of samples from a large number of normal adults. Of note is the degree of variation encountered in these values. This is indicated by the large standard deviations seen in spite of the fact that the values were collected in a single centre using standardized reagents and methods of data collection. This variation between normal individuals makes it difficult to identify perturbations in circulating progenitor numbers in specific patients unless these are very marked, or serial measurements are performed.

LTC-IC measurements have also been applied to normal peripheral blood (Dooley & Law, 1992; Udomsakdi *et al.*, 1992b, c). For these, it has proven necessary to remove the circulating T cells (e.g. by rosetting with sheep erythrocytes) from the test cell suspension prior to initiating the LTC, otherwise spontaneous outgrowth of EBV-transformed B lymphocytes frequently occurs and this obscures the detection of clonogenic myeloid cells derived from the input LTC-IC. As seen by a comparison of the data shown in Tables 3.1 and 3.2, the ratio of LTC-IC to clonogenic cells in the blood ($\sim 1:50$) is somewhat lower than the ratio of these two cell types in the marrow ($\sim 1:20$). No differences in the proliferative or differentiative potential of LTC-IC from normal blood or marrow sources have been identified (Sutherland *et al.*, 1989; Udomsakdi *et al.*, 1992b, c), although the marrow LTC-IC appear to include a larger proportion of cells with activated features (Udomsakdi *et al.*, 1992a). In contrast, circulating clonogenic cells differ significantly from their clonogenic counterparts in normal marrow. A higher proportion of the clonogenic progenitors in the blood belong to the more primitive categories and none appears to be proliferating (Eaves & Eaves, 1987; Udomsakdi *et al.*, 1992c) (see also Table 3.2). In fact, phenotypically, the clonogenic cells in the circulation closely resemble marrow LTC-IC, although they can be partially separated from circulating LTC-IC (Udomsakdi *et al.*, 1992c). At present similar purification strategies applied to marrow or blood cells allow LTC-IC to be enriched up to 2000-fold (Sutherland *et al.*, 1989; Udomsakdi *et al.*, 1991, 1992c). Even so, final purities in excess of a few per cent are not yet achievable.

Conclusions

A variety of cell culture procedures allow primitive human hematopoietic cells to be enumerated following expression of their developmental potential. In many cases these procedures exploit the principle of sequential transfer of cells from one type of culture to another, reflecting the fact that different conditions may be required to optimize the growth of cells at different stages of differentiation. The LTC-IC assay offers a quantitative and widely applicable assay for cells that, by extrapolation from murine studies, appear to overlap with cells able to competitively restore the entire hematopoietic system. Presumably this reflects the production by fibroblasts of unique factors able to support the self-renewal and initial differentiation of these early cells (Sutherland *et al.*, 1993). The utility of LTC-IC assays in predicting the speed of hematologic recovery in recipients of peripheral blood or marrow transplants is unknown. Experience in the mouse would suggest that early hematopoietic recovery in humans is not, in fact, related to the number of LTC-IC transplanted. Rather it may depend on the presence of subtly altered cells no longer detectable as LTC-IC, which may be identified by shorter term *in vitro* assays that, nevertheless, are selective for progenitors of high proliferative potential. The challenge for the future is to identify the molecular basis of these changes in factor responsiveness of very primitive hematopoietic cells and their regulation towards the long-term goal of defining conditions for the controlled amplification of any hematopoietic progenitor cell type of interest.

Acknowledgments

This work was supported by the National Cancer Institute of Canada (NCIC). C.J. Eaves is a Terry Fox Research Scientist of the NCIC. The expert secretarial assistance of Ms C. Kelly is also acknowledged.

28   *C.J. Eaves and A.C. Eaves*

References

Abkowitz, J.L., Linenberger, M.L., Newton, M.A., Shelton, G.H., Ott, R.L. & Guttorp, P. (1990). Evidence for the maintenance of hematopoiesis in a large animal by the sequential activation of stem-cell clones. *Proc. Nat. Acad. Sci. USA*, **87**: 9062–6.

Abrams, R.A., Glaubiger, D., Appelbaum, F.R. & Deisseroth, A.B. (1980). Result of attempted hematopoietic reconstitution using isologous, peripheral blood mononuclear cells: a case report. *Blood*, **56**: 516–20.

Axelrad, A.A. (1990). Some hemopoietic negative regulators. *Exp. Hematol.*, **18**: 143–50.

Baum, C.M., Weissman, I.L., Tsukamoto, A.S. & Buckle, A-M. (1992). Isolation of a candidate human hematopoietic stem-cell population. *Proc. Nat. Acad. Sci. USA*, **89**: 2804–8.

Brecher, G. & Cronkite, E.P. (1951). Post-radiation parabiosis and survival in rats. *Proc. Soc. Exp. Biol. Med.*, **77**: 292–4.

Cashman, J., Eaves, A.C. & Eaves, C.J. (1985). Regulated proliferation of primitive hematopoietic progenitor cells in long-term human marrow cultures. *Blood*, **66**: 1002–5.

Cavins, J.A., Scheer, S.C., Thomas, E.D. & Ferrebee, J.W. (1964). The recovery of lethally irradiated dogs given infusions of autologous leukocytes preserved at −80°C. *Blood*, **23**: 38–43.

Cormack, D. (1976). Time-lapse characterization of erythrocytic colony-forming cells in plasma cultures. *Exp. Hemat.*, **4**: 319–27.

Dexter, T.M. & Spooncer, E. (1987). Growth and differentiation in the hemopoietic system. *Ann. Rev. Cell Biol.*, **3**: 423–41.

Dick, J.E. (1991). Immune-deficient mice as models of normal and leukemic human hematopoiesis. *Cancer Cells*, **3**: 39–48.

Dick, J.E., Magli, M.C., Huszar, D., Phillips, R.A. & Bernstein, A. (1985). Introduction of a selectable gene into primitive stem cells capable of long-term reconstitution of the hemopoietic system of W/Wᵛ mice. *Cell*, **42**: 71–9.

Dooley, D.C. & Law, P. (1992). Detection and quantitation of long-term culture-initiating cells in normal human peripheral blood. *Exp. Hematol.*, **20**: 156–60.

Dowding, C.R. & Gordon, M.Y. (1992). Physical, phenotypic and cytochemical characterisation of stroma-adherent blast colony-forming cells. *Leukemia*, **6**: 347–51.

Eaves, C.J. & Eaves, A.C. (1987). Cell culture studies in CML. In *Chronic Myeloid Leukaemia Bailliere's Clinical Haematology*, ed. J.M. Goldman, vol. 1, no. 4, pp. 931–61. Baillière Tindall, London.

Eaves, C.J., Cashman, J.D. & Eaves, A.C. (1991a). Methodology of long-term culture of human hemopoietic cells. *J. Tissue Culture Methods*, **13**: 55–62.

Eaves, C.J., Cashman, J.D., Sutherland, H.J. *et al.* (1991b). Molecular analysis of primitive hematopoietic cell proliferation control mechanisms. *Ann. NY Acad. Sci.*, **628**: 298–306.

Eaves, C.J., Sutherland, H.J., Udomsakdi, C. *et al.* (1992). The human hematopoietic stem cell in vitro and in vivo. *Blood Cells*, **18**: 301–7.

Epstein, R.B., Graham, T.C. & Buckner, C.D. (1966). Allogeneic marrow engraftment by cross circulation in lethally irradiated dogs. *Blood*, **28**: 692—707.

Fraser, C.C., Szilvassy, S.J., Eaves, C.J. & Humphries, R.K. (1992). Proliferation of totipotent hematopoietic stem cells in vitro with retention of long-term competitive in vivo reconstituting ability. *Proc. Natl. Acad. Sci. USA*, **89**: 1968–72.

Goodman, J.W. & Hodgson, G.S. (1962). Evidence for stem cells in the peripheral blood of mice. *Blood*, **19**: 702–14.

Jandl, J.H. (1987). Physiology of red cells. In *Blood –Textbook of Hematology*, pp. 49–109. Little, Brown and Company, Boston/Toronto.

Jones, R.J., Celano, P., Sharkis, S.J. & Sensenbrenner, L.L. (1989). Two phases of engraftment established by serial bone marrow transplantation in mice. *Blood*, **73**: 397–401.

Jones, R.J., Wagner, J.E., Celano, P., Zicha, M.S. & Sharkis, S.J. (1990). Separation of pluripotent haematopoietic stem cells from spleen colony-forming cells. *Nature*, **347**: 188–9.

Keller, G. & Snodgrass, R. (1990). Life span of multipotential hematopoietic stem cells in vivo. *J. Exp. Med.*, **171**: 1407–18.

Kyoizumi, S., Baum, C.M., Kaneshima, H., McCune, J.M., Yee, E.J. & Namikawa, R. (1992). Implantation and maintenance of functional human bone marrow in SCID-hu mice. *Blood*, **79**: 1704–11.

Lapidot, T., Pflumio, F., Doedens, M., Murdoch, B., Williams, D.E. & Dick, J.E. (1992). Cytokine stimulation of multilineage hematopoiesis from immature human cells engrafted in SCID mice. *Science*, **255**: 1137–41.

Leary, A.G., Zeng, H.Q., Clark, S.C. & Ogawa, M. (1992). Growth factor requirements for survival in G_0 and entry into the cell cycle of primitive human hemopoietic progenitors. *Proc. Natl. Acad. Sci. USA*, **89**: 4013–17.

Lemischka, I.R., Raulet, D.H. & Mulligan, R.C. (1986). Developmental potential and dynamic behavior of hematopoietic stem cells. *Cell*, **45**: 917–27.

McCulloch, E.A. & Till, J.E. (1960). The radiation sensitivity of normal mouse bone marrow cells, determined by quantitative marrow transplantation into irradiated mice. *Radiat. Res.*, **13**: 115–125.

McNiece, I.K., Stewart, F.M., Deacon, D.M. *et al.* (1989). Detection of a human CFC with a high proliferative potential. *Blood*, **74**: 609–12.

Moore, M.A.S. (1991). Clinical implications of positive and negative hematopoietic stem cell regulators. *Blood*, **78**: 1–19.

Namikawa, R., Weilbaecher, K.N., Kaneshima, H., Yee, E.J. & McCune, J.M. (1990). Long-term human hematopoiesis in the SCID-hu mouse. *J. Exp. Med.*, **172**: 1055–63.

Ploemacher, R.E. & Brons, N.H.C. (1988). Isolation of hemopoietic stem cell subsets from murine bone marrow: II. Evidence for an early precursor of day-12 CFU-S and cells associated with radioprotective ability. *Exp. Hematol.*, **16**: 27–32.

Ploemacher, R.E. & Brons, R.H.C. (1989). Separation of CFU-S from primitive cells responsible for reconstitution of the bone marrow hemopoietic stem cell compartment following irradiation: evidence for a pre-CFU-S cell. *Exp. Hematol.*, **17**: 263–6.

Ploemacher, R.E., van Der Sluijs, J.P., Voerman, J.S.A. & Brons, N.H.C. (1989). An in vitro limiting-dilution assay of long-term repopulating hematopoietic stem cells in the mouse. *Blood*, **74**: 2755–63.

Ploemacher, R.E., van der Sluijs, J.P., van Beurden, C.A.J., Baert, M.R.M. & Chan, P.L. (1991). Use of limiting-dilution type long-term marrow cultures in frequency analysis of marrow-repopulating and spleen colony-forming hematopoietic stem cells in the mouse. *Blood*, **78**: 2527–33.

Siminovitch, L., McCulloch, E.A. & Till, J.E. (1963). The distribution of colony-forming cells among spleen colonies. *J. Comp. Cellular Physiol.*, **62**: 327–36.

Slovick, F.T., Abboud, C.N., Brennan, J.K. & Lichtman, M.A. (1984). Survival of granulocytic progenitors in the nonadherent and adherent compartments of human long-term marrow cultures. *Exp. Hematol.*, **12**: 327–38.

Smith, L.G., Weissman, I.L. & Heimfeld, S. (1991). Clonal analysis of hematopoietic stem-cell differentiation in vivo. *Proc. Natl. Acad. Sci. USA*, **88**: 2788–92.

Srour, E.F., Zanjani, E.D., Brandt, J.E. *et al.* (1992). Sustained human hematopoiesis in sheep transplanted in utero during early gestation with fractionated adult human bone marrow cells. *Blood*, **79**: 1404–12.

Storb, R., Graham, T.C., Epstein, R.B., Sale, G.E. & Thomas, E.D. (1977). Demonstration of hemopoietic stem cells in the peripheral blood of baboons by cross circulation. *Blood*, **50**: 537–42.

Sutherland, H.J., Eaves, A.C. & Eaves, C.J. (1991a). Quantitative assays for human hemopoietic progenitor cells. In *Bone Marrow Processing and Purging: A Practical Guide*, ed. A.P. Gee, pp. 155–71. CRC Press, Boca Raton, FL.

Sutherland, H.J., Eaves, C.J., Eaves, A.C., Dragowska, W. & Lansdorp, P.M. (1989). Characterization and partial purification of human marrow cells capable of initiating long-term hematopoiesis in vitro. *Blood*, **74**: 1563–70.

Sutherland, H.J., Eaves, C.J., Lansdorp, P.M., Thacker, J.D. & Hogge, D.E. (1991b). Differential regulation of primitive human hematopoietic cells in long-term cultures maintained on genetically engineered murine stromal cells. *Blood*, **78**: 666–72.

Sutherland, H.J., Hogge, D.E., Cook, D. & Eaves, C.J. (1993). Alternative mechanisms with and without steel factor support primitive human hematopoiesis. *Blood* **81**: 1465–70.

Sutherland, H.J., Lansdorp, P.M., Henkelman, D.H., Eaves, A.C. & Eaves, C.J. (1990). Functional characterization of individual human hematopoietic stem cells cultured at limiting dilution on supportive marrow stromal layers. *Proc. Natl. Acad. Sci. USA*, **87**: 3584–8.

Szilvassy, S.J., Fraser, C.C., Eaves, C.J., Lansdorp, P.M., Eaves, A.C. & Humphries, R.K. (1989a). Retrovirus-mediated gene transfer to purified hemopoietic stem cells with long-term lympho-myelopoietic repopulating ability. *Proc. Natl. Acad. Sci. USA*, **86**: 8798–802.

Szilvassy, S.J., Humphries, R.K., Lansdorp, P.M., Eaves, A.C. & Eaves, C.J. (1990). Quantitative assay for totipotent reconstituting hematopoietic stem cells by a competitive repopulation strategy. *Proc. Natl. Acad. Sci USA*, **87**: 8736–40.

Szilvassy, S.J., Lansdorp, P.M., Humphries, R.K., Eaves, A.C. & Eaves, C.J. (1989b). Isolation in a single step of a highly enriched murine hematopoietic stem cell population with competitive long-term repopulating ability. *Blood*, **74**: 930–9.

Till, J.E. & McCulloch, E.A. (1961). A direct measurement of the radiation sensitivity of normal mouse bone marrow cells. *Radiat. Res.*, **14**: 213–22.

Turhan, A.G., Humphries, R.K., Phillips, G.L., Eaves, A.C. & Eaves, C.J. (1989). Clonal hematopoiesis demonstrated by X-linked DNA polymorphisms after allogeneic bone marrow transplantation. *N. Engl. J. Med.*, **320**: 1655–61.

Udomsakdi, C., Eaves, C.J., Lansdorp, P.M. & Eaves, A.C. (1992a). Phenotypic heterogeneity of primitive leukemic hematopoietic cells in patients with chronic myeloid leukemia (CML). *Blood*, **80**: 2522–30.

Udomsakdi, C., Eaves, C.J., Sutherland, H.J. & Lansdorp, P.M. (1991). Separation of functionally distinct subpopulations of primitive human hematopoietic cells using rhodamine-123. *Exp. Hemat.*, **19**: 338–42.

Udomsakdi, C. Eaves, C.J., Swolin, B., Reid, D.S., Barnett, M.J. & Eaves, A.C. (1992b). Rapid decline of chronic myeloid leukemic cells in long-term culture due to a defect at the leukemic stem cell level. *Proc. Natl. Acad. Scie. USA*, **89**: 6192–6.

Udomsakdi, C., Lansdorp, P.M., Hogge, D.E., Reid, D.S., Eaves, A.C. & Eaves, C.J. (1992c). Characterization of primitive hematopoietic cells in normal human peripheral blood. *Blood*, **78**: 1041–6.

Wu, A.M., Till, J.E., Siminovitch, L. & McCulloch, E.A. (1968). Cytological evidence for a relationship between normal hematopoietic colony-forming cells and cells of the lymphoid system. *J. Exp. Med.*, **127**: 455–64.

4

Isolating stem and progenitor cells

W. BENSINGER

Introduction

Since the original demonstration in mice that the infusion of syngeneic marrow could protect against the lethal effects of total body irradiation, investigators have searched for the cell or cells contained in marrow that are responsible for hematopoietic reconstitution. In recent years, with rapid expansion of applications for marrow transplants, the search for these cells has become urgent. The ability to isolate cell(s) responsible for hematopoietic reconstitution would help our understanding of the physiology of hematopoiesis. Isolated stem cells could be used to facilitate gene transfer studies and their clinical application. Purified stem cells that are free of tumor cells would provide an excellent alternative to marrow purging. Such an approach may be especially useful in the application of purified stem cells to autologous transplants for patients with malignant diseases that involve the stem cell, such as chronic myelogenous leukemia (CML), where there is evidence of the coexistence of a very small population of nonmalignant stem cells. Mature T cells are not contained in stem cell isolates and therefore these cells could potentially be used successfully in allotransplants. Starting with a highly purified stem cell concentrate it may be possible to develop *in vitro* techniques for the culture and propagation of large numbers of stem cells or to improve on existing methodologies for *ex vivo* purging of marrow utilizing long-term marrow cultures.

What is a stem cell?

The exact nature of the cell or cells that contribute to hematopoietic reconstitution is unknown. Operationally, stem cells may be defined as cells capable of self-renewal and differentiation into one or all of the mature cells found in peripheral blood. A more thorough discussion of the characteristics of stem cells is contained in Chapter 3. Methods to isolate stem cells must rely on physical properties that can distinguish these cells from other cells contained in marrow or blood. Success in stem cell purification has been hampered by the lack of assays for pluripotent stem cells. Until recently, it was known only that stem cells were found in the mononuclear fraction prepared from marrow and had a morphology resembling blast cells (Fitchen *et al.*, 1981). Early attempts to purify stem cells utilized density gradient separation or elutriation of mononuclear cells (Visser & Bol, 1981; Ellis *et al.*, 1984; deWitte *et al.*, 1986). Investigators have subsequently discovered that a monoclonal antibody raised against the leukemia cell line KG-1A reacted with 1–2% of mononuclear cells in human marrow that gave rise to virtually all hematopoietic colonies and their precursors detectable *in vitro* (Civin *et al.*, 1984). The antigen defined by this antibody was designated CD34. Several other monoclonal antibodies have been raised against the CD34 antigen, greatly facilitating efforts to purify stem cells (Andrews *et al.*, 1986; Watt *et al.*, 1987). The proof that CD34$^+$ cells contained stem cells required the demonstration in primates that these cells alone were necessary and sufficient for hematopoietic recovery after marrow ablative total body irradiation (Berenson *et al.*, 1988). Without a unique marker to identify cells that were reinfused from residual host cells even this experiment did not prove that the infused CD34$^+$ cells were responsible for long-term hematopoietic reconstitution. It is known, furthermore, that the CD34$^+$ fraction of marrow contains a heterogeneous population of cells of which only a few have the important stem cell property of extensive self-renewal (Bernstein *et al.*, 1991). Efforts to further purify stem cells have focused on the separation of CD34$^+$ cells which are devoid of other cell surface antigens; so-called 'lineage negative' (lin$^-$) cells, and cells that are in G_0 and are resistant to 5-fluorouracil (Andrews *et al.*, 1990; Srour *et al.*, 1991; Terstappen *et al.*, 1991; Bernstein *et al.*, 1991). Studies have demonstrated that these cells have no ability to form colonies directly in short-term *in vitro* assays but with appropriate stimulation using preformed stromal layers or combinations of cytokines can give rise to multilineage colonies. Recently it has been possible to show that allogeneic CD34$^+$ marrow cells depleted of T and B cells are capable of short-term and long-term (up to 1 year) hematopoietic reconstitution in primates (Andrews *et al.*, unpublished data). It has been estimated that the actual frequency of true stem cells in the marrow ranges from $1/10^4$ to $2/10^5$ cells.

W. Bensinger

Techniques for stem cell isolation

Density gradient centrifugation and elutriation techniques have been used to isolate low-density nucleated marrow cells depleted of lymphocytes and with enriched proportions of progenitors detectable *in vitro* (Visser & Bol, 1981; Ellis *et al.*, 1984; Humblet *et al.*, 1988; Wagner *et al.*, 1990). Since these methods were developed using *in vitro* progenitor assays as indirect measurements of stem cells, it is unknown whether the true pluripotent stem cell copurifies. Recent data in mice suggest that using counterflow elutriation, the true pluripotent hematopoietic stem cell can be separated from not only *in vitro* colony-forming cells but also both day 8 and day 12 CFU-S (Jones *et al.*, 1990). Further studies using this fraction of cells should provide important insights into stem cell function. Such a technique probably is not useful for clinical studies as these mice required a temporary surrogate graft in order to survive the long period of time required for the stem cells to function. This makes elutriation or density gradient procedures suitable for volume reduction, red cell depletion, T cell depletion or further purging procedures but they do not provide adequate enrichment or discrimination of stem cells and progenitors from non-stem cells, including tumor cells.

The most widely used device for stem cell separation is the fluorescence activated cell sorter (FACS). Cells labeled with an anti-CD34 antibody may be sorted directly or counterstained with common T and B cell lineage antibodies to provide CD34$^+$ lin$^-$ cells. A preparation of the same cells must be stained with irrelevant antibodies of the same class or isotype to establish negative threshold fluorescence parameters for sorting the cells that are positive. Clearly, FACS has the capability to provide cells most homogeneous for a given antigen specificity. The limited capacity of FACS limits its utility to cell separation for *in vitro* or small animal studies. This usually requires a preenrichment step such as density gradient separation often with immunorosetting or removal of plastic adherent cells (Andrews *et al.*, 1990; Lansdorp *et al.*, 1990; Terstappen *et al.*, 1991). Without preenrichment of the desired population very long sorting times that require many hours are needed in order to obtain adequate numbers of cells.

Immunorosetting methodology with red cells, floating beads or magnetic beads have been widely applied to marrow manipulation, largely to deplete cell populations for the elimination of T cells, tumor cells or the indirect enrichment of progenitors (Spangrude *et al.*, 1988; Andrews *et al.*, 1990; Gabbianelli *et al.*, 1990; Wormmeester *et al.*, 1990; Terstappen *et al.*, 1991). Immunomagnetic beads have been the popularly used approach for the depletion of certain cell subsets from marrow. One or more antibodies of the same isotype are incubated with the cells of interest. Immunomagnetic microbeads coated with an isotype-specific antiglobulin are mixed with the cells in a ratio of 0.5–5.0 microspheres per cell and incubated. The undesired cells are then separated by holding them in a fixed portion of the container using magnets. The desired cells are then free from both specific cells and any unbound magnetic beads.

When used for depletion this approach is relatively easy and reproducible. Some investigators have used immunomagnetic beads to deplete not only tumor cells but the majority of lin⁻ cells from marrow. The remaining cells are highly enriched for progenitors. Several groups have successfully utilized this approach as an indirect method of progenitor enrichment for *in vitro* and animal studies. In fact, the most purified cells obtained to date have utilized multiple methodologies including Ficoll and Percoll, immunomagnetic beads, and/or FACS (Koizumi *et al.*, 1985; Spangrude *et al.*, 1988; Gabbianelli *et al.*, 1990). The ability to perform these manipulations on the quantities of cells necessary for human studies remains to be determined.

Although it has been possible to demonstrate effective enrichment for stem cells using immunomagnetic beads for positive selection on small amounts of marrow, problems with scale-up have prevented the clinical application of this methodology (Civin *et al.*, 1990; Egeland & Gaudernack, 1992). A major drawback in the use of immunomagnetic beads for positive selection has been the inability to detach the beads from cells. Enzymes such as chymopapain have been utilized for bead detachment but again the ability to scale up this system remains to be determined.

We have utilized an avidin-biotin immunoadsorption column for stem cell isolation. This technique relies on the very high affinity between the protein avidin and the vitamin biotin, which has an association constant up to 10^5 higher than most antigen–antibody interactions (Jasiewicz *et al.*, 1976; Basch *et al.*, 1983; Wormmeester *et al.*, 1984). Avidin is covalently linked to polyacrylamide beads which are sterilized and placed into glass or plastic columns. Marrow buffy coat is washed and incubated with an anti-CD34 antibody. The marrow is washed again and incubated with a secondary antibody that has been biotinylated (goat anti-mouse IgG). Labelled cells are rapidly passed down the avidin column. After the column has been washed, adherent cells are removed by gentle agitation.

We have used this technique to process 28 marrows from patients with neuroblastoma or breast cancer. The results of enrichment are shown in Table 4.1. These results suggest the feasibility of this approach but

Table 4.1. *CD34 enrichment of marrow*

| Number of procedures | Cell recovery | Purity | CD34 progenitor enrichment[a] | |
			CFU-GM (*n* = 18)	LTMC (*n* = 14)
28	1.07% (0.14–2.48)	65% (35–92)	30.7 (0.9–128.9)	79.8 (22–180)

[a]Short-term *in vitro* colony-forming unit-granulocyte/macrophage (CFU-GM) and long-term marrow cultures (LTMC) were used to calculate progenitor enrichment. CFU-GM progenitor enrichment was calculated by dividing the number of colonies generated per 10^5 cells plated in the CD34$^+$ fraction by the number of colonies per 10^5 cells plated in the unselected marrows. LTMC progenitor enrichment was calculated in the same way using all CFU-GM generated in weeks 2–6 in culture per 4×10^6 cells initially plated.

problems with variability and reproducibility remain. Measurement of short-term progenitors suggest that enrichment, on average, is not as great as for progenitors detectable in the long-term marrow culture. One explanation for this disparity, other than simply assay variability, is that more mature and thus more committed progenitors display a lower CD34 antigen density, making them less likely to bind to an immunoaffinity column.

We have used antibody 12.8 but there is no reason why other antibodies cannot be used (Berenson *et al.*, 1987a; Tassi *et al.*, 1991). In a dog model we utilized an anti-Ia antibody to separate marrow repopulating cells (Berenson *et al.*, 1987b). Other studies using directly biotinylated 12.8 have not shown any major differences in recovery. These cells are functionally capable of hematopoietic reconstitution in canines, primates and humans (Berenson *et al.*, 1987a, 1988, 1991). Although it is clear that antibodies and avidin remain bound to the surface, the cells are able to function *in vivo*. This is not surprising in light of earlier studies in mice demonstrating that avidin-coated cells had superior recovery of CFU-S compared with cells coated only with antibodies (Bauman *et al.*, 1985). These CD34-enriched cells have been infused into 13 patients following high dose chemotherapy with or without total body irradiation. All evaluable patients have had hematopoietic reconstitution (Bensinger *et al.*, 1992).

In preliminary studies it appears possible to separate large numbers of CD34-enriched cells from the blood of patients undergoing cytokine-mobilized blood stem cell collections. Using a similar avidin-biotin immunoadsorption device we have been able to collect 1×10^6 to 3×10^6 nucleated cells from a starting number of 500×10^6 cells (0.5% recovery) that were 45% (median) CD34 positive and were enriched 40–100-fold for CFU-GM/10^5 cells plated. More studies are underway to determine the properties of these cells.

In a related methodology investigators have developed antibody–antibody complexes that bind specifically both to cells of interest and to glass beads. The desired cells can be eluted by disruption of the antibody complex with dithiothreitol (Thomas *et al.*, 1989). This approach in theory should result in cells more highly purified than those obtained by immunoadsorption alone, as cells must not only be specifically bound but specifically eluted. Preliminary results in relatively small samples are promising, although once again the ability to scale up this method has not been demonstrated and no data were presented on the yield of this system.

Other technology to isolate stem cells has relied on a panning technique in which CD34$^+$/HLA DR$^-$ cells were isolated using multilayer plastic containers with an anti-CD34 antibody linked to the surface. The technique as described required several preenrichment steps including density gradient centrifugation, elutriation and removal of soybean agglutinin positive cells (Wagner *et al.*, 1992). The final cell preparation was 20–59-fold enriched for progenitors, but it is difficult to assess the final yield of CD34$^+$ cells.

Critical issues and problems in stem cell transplants

Exactly what cells can and should be isolated for stem cell transplants? The requirements necessary for the isolation of stem cells depends on the proposed use. In the case of clinical application for autologous transplants, the ideal stem cell concentrate should be capable of providing reconstitution that is as rapid as whole, unmodified marrow. To satisfy this requirement, first, the concentrate should contain not only pluripotent stem cells but more committed cells capable of maturing to all the necessary blood elements within a few days. Second, the cells to be reinfused should be free from any contaminating tumor cells. As *in vitro* data suggest that CD34 antigen positive cells contain both committed and less mature progenitors, any selection system utilizing any of the available anti-CD34 antibodies should satisfy the first requirement. Clearly attempts to purify CD34$^+$ lin$^-$ cells from marrow or blood would likely be counterproductive to the aim of early hematopoietic reconstitution, as these cells would require a relatively long time to begin producing differentiated, mature progeny.

With the increased emphasis on peripheral blood stem cell transplants, any stem cell selection procedure should be able to capture the majority of

Table 4.2. *Avidin-biotin immunoadsorption of CD34⁺ marrow cells
followed by FACS sorting of CD34⁺ cells*

Procedure	Total no. $\times 10^6$	Absolute no.		Efficiency (%)
		CD34$^+$ cells (%)	of CD34$^+$ cells $\times 10^6$	
Start	3600	5.8	209	
ABIA	132	61.0	81	39
FACS	19	84.9	16	20

ABIA, avidin-biotin immunoadsorption; FACS, fluorescence activated cell sorter.

cells that contribute to engraftment in a given collection. This is an important issue because it is not known whether the cells collected in peripheral blood that contribute to engraftment have the same characteristics as stem cells found in marrow. It may be, for example, that the CD34 antigen is not expressed on all stem cells found in blood or that cytokine mobilization may alter the antigenic phenotype of these cells. These important questions need to be answered before CD34 selection is widely applied to peripheral blood. As these issues are addressed, it will be necessary to continue the development of technology capable of handling the often massive numbers (up to 10 times more) of cells collected for blood stem cell transplants.

Another problem related to stem cell isolation methods is low recovery of stem cells. All the available methodologies for stem cell isolation and purification procedures result in enrichment of progenitors but also substantial losses of the original numbers of stem cells, as measured by progenitors or CD34 antigen expression, that were present in the original unmodified marrows. The avidin-biotin immunoadsorption system, for example, typically recovers only 30–60% of the absolute number of CD34⁺ cells that were present in the original unmodified marrow. Other technologies have similar or greater losses. Cell sorters, for example, are no more efficient in terms of cell yield than other currently available technologies. Cell losses with FACS typically exceed 50%. Table 4.2 lists the number of cells, purity, absolute number of CD34⁺ cells and percentage recovery of CD34⁺ cells from an experiment using an avidin-biotin immunoadsorption column to purify CD34⁺ cells from baboon marrow followed by sorting of the column-enriched cells by FACS. Avidin-biotin immunoadsorption recovered 39% of the available CD34⁺ cells in the unselected marrow. FACS sorting recovered 20% of the CD34⁺ cells available after CD34 enrichment using avidin-biotin immunoadsorption. This recovery holds true regardless of the technique used to preenrich cells for CD34 prior to FACS sorting. It should also be mentioned that the sorting of the 132×10^6 cells to yield 19×10^6 cells required more than 12 continuous hours of FACS time. Clearly, methodological advances must include increasing the efficiency of stem cell recovery especially when applied to the treatment of patients with malignant disease who often have reduced stem function or numbers.

The CD34 antigen is not found on tumor cells from patients with breast cancer, neuroblastoma, lymphomas and multiple myeloma, making patients with these malignancies suitable for treatment. Theoretically, stem cell isolates using CD34 selection from patients with these disorders should be tumor free. In practical application this is not the case. Using the avidin-biotin system as an example the average purity of CD34 enriched cells using the data presented earlier is only 65%. This means that one-third of the cells are neither stem cells nor progenitors. While analysis reveals that the majority of these contaminating cells are granulocytes, analysis for residual breast cancer cells after CD34 enrichment indicates that some breast cancer cells remain. We have used immunocytokeratin (ICC) staining to look for residual ICC$^+$ cells in marrow processed for CD34 enrichment. In some CD34-enriched samples ICC$^+$ cells are still detectable. The clinical significance of these positive cells in terms of their potential to cause relapse is uncertain, especially in light of the very high relapse rate attributable to the failure to eradicate host disease. A goal of stem cell isolation procedures should be to eliminate all tumor cells.

Will stem cell isolates result in a higher cure rate for patients with malignant disease? There is no inherent reason why highly purified stem cells should be better able to cure malignant disease than whole marrow or peripheral blood. In addition, as previously noted, the value of completely tumor-free marrow is uncertain because most relapses are the result of inadequate conditioning regimens and there is data from patients with acute nonlymphocytic leukemia to suggest that complete eradication of all leukemia cells is not a necessary prerequisite for cure. It is likely that infusions of purified stem cells per se will probably not measurably contribute to cure of patients.

Are stem cell transplants needed? The same argument has prevailed over autologous transplants for many years. There are few studies in patients that demonstrate the necessity for marrow transplants to achieve long-term hematopoietic reconstitution. The value of stem cell isolates is currently only promising and is yet to be proven. Other technologies such as more

efficient gene transfer and *in vitro* stem cell propagation must be developed
to make full use of isolation techniques. The use of allogeneic stem cell
isolates to cure nonmalignant diseases has theoretical appeal because of the
potential for elimination of the risk of graft-versus-host disease. Certainly,
as a research tool, stem cell purification has proven unique value.
Considerable progress in this field will undoubtedly continue.

Acknowledgements

This work is supported by grants CA 18029 and CA 47748.

References

Andrews, R.G., Singer, J.W. & Bernstein, I.D. (1986). Monoclonal antibody 12.8
    recognizes a 115-kd molecule present on both unipotent and multipotent
    hematopoietic colony-forming cells and their precursors. *Blood*, **67**: 842–5.
Andrews, R.G., Singer, J.W. & Bernstein, I.D. (1990). Human hematopoietic
    precursors in long term culture: single CD34[+] cells that lack detectable T, B,
    and myeloid antigens produce multiple colony-forming cells when cultured
    with marrow stromal cells. *J. Exp. Med.*, **172**: 355–8.
Basch, R.S., Berman, J.W. & Lakow, E. (1983). Cell separation using positive
    immunoselective techniques. *J. Immunol. Methods*, **56**: 269–80.
Bauman, J.G.J., Mulder, A.H. & van den Engh, G.J. (1985). Effect of surface
    antigen labelling on spleen colony formation: comparison of the indirect
    immunofluorescence and the biotin-avidin methods. *Exp. Hematol*, **13**: 760–7.
Bensinger, W.I., Berenson, R.J., Andrews, R.G. *et al.* (1992). Engraftment after
    infusion of CD34 enriched marrow cells. *Int. J. Cell Cloning*, **10** (suppl. 1):
    35–7.
Berenson, R.J., Andrews, R.G., Bensinger, W.I. *et al.* (1988). Antigen CD34[+]
    marrow cells engraft lethally irradiated baboons. *J. Clin. Invest.*, **81**: 951–5.
Berenson, R.J., Bensinger, W.I., Andrews, R.G. *et al.* (1987a). Hematopoietic stem
    cell transplants. In *Recent Advances in Leukemia and Lymphoma, UCLA
    Symposia on Molecular and Cellular Biology, New Series*, ed. R.P. Gale &
    D.W. Golde, vol. 61, pp. 527–33. Alan R. Liss, New York.
Berenson, R.J., Bensinger, W.I., Hill, R.S. *et al.* (1991). Engraftment after infusion
    of CD34[+] marrow cells in patients with breast cancer or neuroblastoma.
    Blood, **77**: 1717–22.
Berenson, R.J., Bensinger, W.I., Kalamasz, D. *et al.* (1987b). Engraftment of dogs
    with Ia-positive marrow cells isolated by avidin-biotin immunoadsorption.
    Blood, **69**: 1363–7.
Bernstein, I.D., Andrews, R.G. & Zsebo, K.M. (1991). Recombinant human stem
    cell factor enhances the formation of colonies by CD34[+] and CD34[+] lin[−]
    cells, and the generation of colony-forming cell progeny from CD34[+] lin[−]
    cells cultured with interleukin-3 (IL-3), granulocyte-macrophage
    colony-stimulating factor (GM-CSF), or granulocyte colony stimulating factor
    (G-CSF). *Blood*, **77**: 2316–21.
Civin, C.I., Strauss, L.C., Brovall, C., Fackler, M.J., Schwartz, J.F. & Shaper, J.H.
    (1984). Antigenic analysis of hematopoiesis. III. A hematopoietic progenitor
    cell surface antigen defined by a monoclonal antibody raised against KG-1a
    cells. *J. Immunol.*, **133**: 157–65.

Civin, C.I., Strauss, L.C., Fackler, M.J., Trischmann, T.M., Wiley, J.M. & Loken, M.R. (1990). Positive stem cell selection: basic science. *Prog. Clin. Biol. Res.*, **333**: 387–401

DeWitte, T., Hoogenhout, J., dePauw, B. *et al.* (1986). Depletion of donor lymphocytes by counterflow centrifugation successfully prevents acute graft-versus-host disease in matched allogeneic marrow transplantation. *Blood*, **67**: 1302–8.

Egeland, T. & Gaudernack, G. (1992). A new series of CD34 monoclonal antibodies designed for immunomagnetic isolation of human and rhesus monkey bone marrow stem cells. *Bone Marrow Transplant.*, **190** (D204), abstract.

Ellis, W.M., Georgiou, G.M., Roberton, D.M. & Johnson, G.R. (1984). The use of discontinuous percoll gradients to separate populations of cells from human bone marrow and peripheral blood. *J. Immunol. Methods*, **66**: 9–16.

Fitchen, J.H., Foon, K.A. & Cline, M.J. (1981). The antigenic characteristics of hematopoietic stem cells. *N. Engl. J. Med.*, **305**: 17–24.

Gabbianelli, M., Sargiacomo, M., Pelosi, E., Testa, U., Isacchi, G. & Peschle, C. (1990). 'Pure' human hematopoietic progenitors: permissive action of basic fibroblast growth factor. *Science*, **249**: 1561–4.

Humblet, Y., Lefebvre, P., Jacques, J.L. *et al.* (1988). Concentration of bone marrow progenitor cells by separation on a percoll gradient using the haemonetics model 30. *Bone Marrow Transplant.*, **3**: 63–7.

Jasiewicz, M.L., Schoenberg, D.R. & Mueller, G.C. (1976). Selective retrieval of biotin-labelled cells using immobilized avidin. *Exp. Cell Res.*, **100**: 213–17.

Jones, R.J., Wagner, J.E., Celano, P., Zicha, M.S. & Sharkis, S.J. (1990). Separation of pluripotent haematopoietic stem cells from spleen colony-forming cells. *Nature*, **347**: 188–9.

Koizumi, S., Fine, R.L., Curt, G.A. & Griffin, J.D. (1985). Enrichment of myeloid progenitor cells from normal human bone marrow using an immune-rosette technique. *Exp. Hematol.*, **13**: 560–5.

Lansdorp, P.M., Sutherland, H.J. & Eaves, C.J. (1990). Selective expression of CD45 isoforms on functional subpopulations of $CD34^+$ hemopoietic cells from human bone marrow. *J. Exp. Med.*, **172**: 363–6.

Spangrude, G.J., Heimfeld, S. & Weissman, I.L. (1988). Purification and characterization of mouse hematopoietic stem cells. *Science*, **241**: 58–62.

Srour, E.F., Brandt, J.E., Briddell, R.A., Leemhuis, T., van Besien, K. & Hoffman, R. (1991). Human $CD34^+$ HLA-DR-bone marrow cells contain progenitor cells capable of self-renewal, multilineage differentiation, and long-term *in vitro* hematopoiesis. *Blood Cells*, **17**: 287–95.

Tassi, C., Fortuna, A., Bontadini, A., Lemoli, R.M., Gobbi, M. & Tazzari, P.L. (1991). CD34 or S313 positive cells selection by avidin-biotin immunoadsorption. *Haematologica*, **76**: 41–3.

Terstappen, L.W.M.M., Huang, S., Safford, M., Lansdorp, P.M. & Loken, M.R. (1991). Sequential generations of hematopoietic colonies derived from single nonlineage-committed $CD34^+$ $CD38^-$ progenitor cells. *Blood*, **77**: 1218–27.

Thomas, T.E., Sutherland, H.J. & Lansdorp, P.M. (1989). Specific binding and release of cells from beads using cleavable tetrameric antibody complexes. *J. Immunol. Methods*, **120**: 221–31.

Visser, J.W.M. & Bol, S.J.L. (1981). A two-step procedure for obtaining 80-fold enriched suspensions of murine pluripotent hemopoietic stem cells. *Stem Cells*, **1**: 240–9.

Wagner, J., Lebkowski, J., Fahey, S. & Okarma, T. (1992). Isolation and enrichment of primitive CD34$^+$/HLA-DR−human hematopoietic stem cells by counterflow elutriation followed by a soybean agglutinin depletion and CD34$^+$ positive selection. *Bone Marrow Transplant.*, **216** (D211), abstract.

Wagner, J.E., Santos, G.W., Noga, S.J. *et al.* (1990). Bone marrow graft engineering by counterflow centrifugal elutriation: results of a phase I–II clinical trial. *Blood,* **75**: 1370.

Watt, S.M., Karhi, K., Gatter, K. *et al.* (1987). Distribution and epitope analysis of the cell membrane glycoprotein (HPCA-1) associated with human hemopoietic progenitor cells. *Leukemia,* **1**: 417–26.

Wormmeester, J., Stiekema, F. & De Groot, C. (1990). Immunoselective cell separation. *Methods Enzymol.*, **184**: 314–19.

Wormmeester, J., Stiekema, F. & De Groot, K. (1984). A simple method for immunoselective cell separation with the avidin-biotin system. *J. Immunol. Methods,* **67**: 389–94.

5

Growth factors and blood stem cells

D.W. MAHER, W.P. SHERIDAN AND A.M. GIANNI

Introduction

The discovery and cloning of the hematopoietic growth factors, or colony-stimulating factors has led to their clinical investigation in a wide range of disorders. During phase I studies of both granulocyte colony-stimulating factor (G-CSF) and granulocyte/macrophage colony-stimulating factor (GM-CSF), rises of up to 100-fold in the number of peripheral blood stem cells were observed (Duhrsen *et al.*, 1988; Socinski *et al.*, 1988; Villeval *et al.*, 1990). The magnitude of this rise was sufficient for harvesting of stem cells after colony-stimulating factor administration and their use for transplantation to be considered. G-CSF and GM-CSF are now licensed for clinical use in most western countries to stimulate neutrophil production after chemotherapy and bone marrow transplantation. In this chapter we review the available data on the use of colony-stimulating factors for blood stem cell mobilization and transplantation.

Effects of hematopoietic growth factors on blood stem cells

Both G-CSF (Duhrsen *et al.*, 1988) and GM-CSF (Socinski *et al.*, 1988; Villeval *et al.*, 1990) administration increase the number of stem cells circulating in the peripheral blood (Figure 5.1). The assays used in these studies were standard 14-day agar cultures of CFU-GM, erythropoietic burst-forming cells (E-BFC) and megakaryocyte colony-forming cells (MK-CFC). Representative results taken from these three studies are shown in Table 5.1 and demonstrated that 8–100-fold increases in stem cell numbers could be induced by G-CSF or GM-CSF. The types of progenitor detectable in peripheral blood included those of all three main lineages and G-CSF and GM-CSF both appeared to mobilize progenitors of each of these lineages proportionately. Although day 14 progenitor assays are not

43

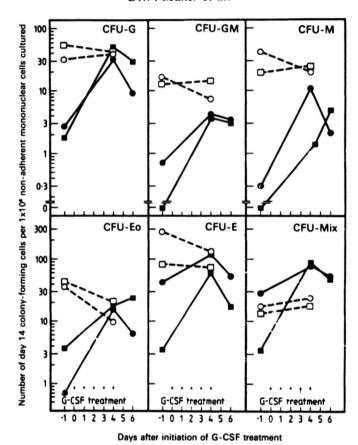

Fig. 5.1. Effect of granulocyte colony-stimulating factor (G-CSF) on circulating and marrow progenitor cells in cancer patients. Closed symbols, solid lines, peripheral blood levels; open symbols, broken lines, bone marrow levels. Squares, 3 μg/kg/day subcutaneously; circles, 10 μg/kg/day intravenously; CFU-G, colony-forming unit (CFU)-granulocyte; CFU-GM, CFU granulocyte/macrophage; CFU-M, CFU macrophage; CFU-Eo, CFU eosinophil; CFU-E, CFU erythropoietic; CFU-Mix, CFU mixed. Reproduced with the permission of Duhrsen *et al.* (1988) and the editor of *Blood*.

a direct measure of long-term reconstituting stem cells the types of progenitor present and the successful use of blood stem cells mobilized post chemotherapy suggested that the cells mobilized by cytokines could also be used in transplants. This concept has been confirmed in mice (Molineux *et al.*, 1990). Blood stem cells mobilized by mouse G-CSF provided stable, long-term hematopoiesis and lymphopoiesis in a sex-mismatched allograft model in this study.

Table 5.1. *Increases in peripheral blood CFU-GM during G-CSF and GM-CSF in phase I studies*

		Level of CFU-GM/ml (S.E.M.)	
Author	CSF, dose, route	Pre-treatment	Day 4 of CSF treatment
Socinski *et al.* (1988)	GM-CSF, 4–64 µg/kg/day by continuous i.v. infusion	36 (15)	469 (144)
Villeval *et al.* (1990)	GM-CSF, 20 µg/kg/day, s.c. injection	100 (150)	880 (1280)
Duhrsen *et al.* (1988)	G-CSF, 10 µg/kg/day, by continuous s.c. infusion	82 (77)	1000 (5000)

CFU, colony-forming unit; CSF, colony-stimulating factor; G, granulocyte; GM, granulocyte/macrophage; i.v., intravenous; s.c., subcutaneous; S.E.M., standard error of mean.

Hematopoietic growth factors after chemotherapy

The use of colony-stimulating factors during recovery from myelotoxic chemotherapy results in amplification of the mobilizing effect induced by chemotherapy alone. It is important to note that not all kinds of chemotherapy are followed by comparable expansion of the circulating stem cell pool. On the basis of limited preclinical as well as clinical data, it would appear that the most marked effect occurs after delivery of severely myelotoxic yet stem cell sparing regimens, resulting in depth of myelosuppression similar to that in the induction phase for acute leukemias (To *et al.*, 1987; Juttner & To, 1991). High dose cyclophosphamide (4–7 g/m²) has been most extensively studied. When administered to patients with non Hodgkin's lymphoma or solid tumors, high dose cyclophosphamide led to an increase in the median concentration of circulating colony-forming unit granulocyte/macrophage (CFU-GM) by approximately 30-fold as compared with basal values (median 149, range 39–329 CFU-GM/ml of peripheral blood) (Gianni *et al.*, 1989a; Juttner & To, 1991).

High dose cyclophosphamide combined with GM-CSF infusion further increased stem cell concentration approximately 100-fold, allowing the harvesting of $\geqslant 30 \times 10^4$ CFU-GM/kg body weight from all 37 patients studied and $\geqslant 50 \times 40^4$ CFU-GM/kg from 86% of patients (Gianni *et al.*, 1993). These very high yields required only two, or at most three, leukaphereses on consecutive days. Comparable results have been obtained

D.W. Maher et al.

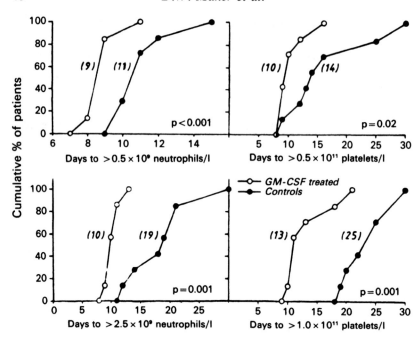

Fig. 5.2. Recovery of peripheral blood neutrophils and platelets after high dose chemoradiotherapy (etoposide, total body irradiation, melphalan). (O) Patients given blood stem cells mobilized with high dose cyclophosphamide and granulocyte/ macrophage colony-stimulating factor (GM-CSF). (●) Patients given blood stem cells mobilized with high dose cyclophosphamide without GM-CSF. Reproduced with the permission of Gianni *et al.* (1989b) and the editor of *The Lancet*.

when G-CSF was substituted for GM-CSF after high dose cyclophosphamide (A.M. Gianni *et al.*, personal communication). Engraftment of neutrophils and platelets was found to be accelerated compared with nonrandomized controls in these studies (Fig. 5.2).

The rise in circulating stem cell numbers after high dose cyclophosphamide or other severely myelosuppressive chemotherapy occurs during the recovery phase of peripheral blood neutrophil and platelet counts, and is brief in duration. It is somewhat hazardous to compare absolute progenitor cell frequency data from different studies because the *in vitro* culture assay for CFU-GM is poorly reproducible and difficult to standardize. For example, the 60-fold increase reported by Socinski *et al.* (1988) for circulating CFU-GM concentration after chemotherapy and GM-CSF infusion, is relative to pretreatment baseline levels of 36, i.e. fourfold lower than the baseline reference value of 149 CFU-GM/ml of Gianni's group. A further confounding factor in comparing reports is the variation in mix of patients with extensive versus limited prior chemotherapy exposure. The colony assay variability problems may be overcome in future by adopting simpler, more reproducible, surrogate assays for stem cells, such as the phenotypic analysis of $CD34^+$ cells using direct flow cytometry of whole peripheral blood (Siena *et al.*, 1989, 1991b).

The combination of colony-stimulating factor and chemotherapy for blood stem cell mobilization has also been reported with the use of chemotherapy considerably less intensive than that of high dose cyclophosphamide. Elias *et al.* (1992a) used GM-CSF during the recovery phase of cycles 3 and 4 of combination chemotherapy in 13 patients with metastatic breast cancer treated with standard doses of cytotoxic agents. Bone marrow was harvested after cycle 2 as a backup. One patient did not undergo high dose chemotherapy and three patients did not engraft after infusion of blood stem cells and required backup bone marrow. The median time to recovery of neutrophils $>0.5 \times 10^9/l$, platelets $>2 \times 10^9/l$ and the duration of hospital stay were all significantly shorter than in 29 historical control patients receiving autologous bone marrow (14 versus 21 days, 12 versus 23 days and 24 versus 38 days, respectively). Gianni *et al.* (personal communication) have recently updated their original series of seven patients (Gianni *et al.*, 1989b). Twenty-five patients, treated with total body irradiation and melphalan, received a combination of bone marrow and GM-CSF-exposed peripheral blood stem cells (followed by postgrafting infusion of GM-CSF in 22 patients). The mean number of days required to achieve $>0.5 \times 10^9$ neutrophils/l was 9 days compared with 11.4 days in seven control patients autografted with bone marrow and circulating stem cells not exposed to GM-CSF. A striking affect on platelet recovery was also confirmed. The time to >50 and $>100 \times 10^9$ platelets/l was significantly shorter compared with controls (11.9 versus 16.9 days and 13.6 versus 24.1 days, respectively). The number of platelet transfusions required was reduced from a mean of 4.1 to 1.5.

Pettengell *et al.* (1992) have presented preliminary data in small groups of patients which suggest that G-CSF during the recovery phase postchemotherapy can also significantly increase the number of blood stem cells. Interestingly, the chemotherapy in this case was the VAPEC-B schedule for lymphoma, which uses relatively low doses of myelotoxic agents on a frequent administration schedule, indicating that intensive myelotoxic chemotherapy is not required for blood stem cell mobilization when G-CSF is also given.

Colony-stimulating factors without chemotherapy

Two phase II studies using GM-CSF (Haas *et al.*, 1990) and two using
G-CSF (Bolwell *et al.*, 1991; Sheridan *et al.*, 1992) mobilized blood stem
cells in autotransplantation have been published or reported in preliminary
form. The study by Haas *et al.* (1990) was in 12 patients who were unable to
have marrow harvested because of hypoplasia or fibrosis after past
chemotherapy or radiotherapy. These patients were given GM-CSF (250
μg/m^2 per day) by continuous intravenous infusion for a median 11.5 days
(range 5–22 days). There was a median 8.5-fold increase in circulating
CFU-GM over baseline with a median CFU-GM content after 10 days of
GM-CSF treatment of 1300/ml peripheral blood. They performed a
median of six leukaphereses in 11 patients with total CFU-GM collected of
6.1–67.6 × 10^5. Six of these patients were autografted with blood stem cells
alone with five of six achieving stable trilineage engraftment, although time
to hematopoietic recovery was slow (median 28.5 days to neutrophils
$> 0.5 \times 10^9$/l and 39 days to platelets $> 20 \times 10^9$/l). These results indicated
that cytokine-mobilized blood stem cells could be successfully used in
patients unsuitable for marrow harvesting. The number of blood stem cells
obtained was low, perhaps reflecting impaired marrow stem cell reserve in
these heavily pretreated patients.

Elias *et al.* (1992b) reported on 13 patients in whom GM-CSF was used
to mobilize blood stem cells. These patients were given GM-CSF (5 μg/kg)
subcutaneously twice daily for 7 days and two leukaphereses were
performed on days 5 and 7. The number of stem cells obtained was not
reported. High dose chemotherapy with ifosfamide, carboplatinum and
etoposide was given, and bone marrow plus blood stem cells were infused.
No GM-CSF was given during the engraftment period. The addition of
blood stem cells mobilized by GM-CSF to autologous bone marrow
infusion significantly shortened the time to neutrophil and platelet recovery
and the total days of hospitalization (17 versus 25 days, 16 versus 18 days
and 27 versus 35 days, respectively) compared with nonrandomized
controls given bone marrow alone.

Sheridan *et al.* (1992) reported a study using G-CSF-mobilized blood
stem cells in pretreated patients with hematologic malignancies. Seventeen
patients were given G-CSF (12 μg/kg, per day) by continuous subcutaneous
infusion for 6 days. Leukaphereses were performed on days 5, 6 and 7.
After high dose chemotherapy with busulphan and cyclophosphamide,
bone marrow and blood stem cells were infused followed by G-CSF (24

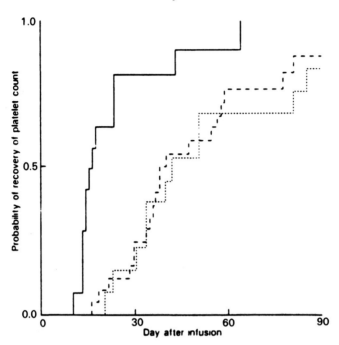

Fig. 5.3. Recovery of peripheral blood platelets after high dose chemotherapy (busulphan and cyclophosphamide). (—) Patients given bone marrow plus granulocyte colony-stimulating factor (G-CSF)-mobilized blood stem cells and post-autograft G-CSF. (– – –) Patients given bone marrow and post-autograft G-CSF. (· · · ·) Patients given bone marrow alone. Overall $p < 0.002$. Reproduced with the permission of Sheridan *et al.* (1992) and the editor of *The Lancet*.

μg/kg per day) by continuous subcutaneous infusion) until neutrophil recovery.

A median 58-fold increase in peripheral blood CFU-GM was obtained with G-CSF therapy enabling $33(\pm 5.7) \times 10^4$ CFU-GM/kg body weight to be collected. Circulating erythroid progenitors rose a median of 24-fold. The addition of blood stem cells to bone marrow had a dramatic effect on the time to platelet recovery, with a reduction from 39 days to 15 days in the median time to reach a platelet count of $50 \times 10^9/l$ and an associated reduction in the requirement for platelet transfusions (Fig. 5.3). These observations have recently been confirmed in a study of similar design (Bolwell *et al.*, 1991).

None of these studies had randomized controls although the results of blood stem cell mobilization are consistent with data in the mouse model for G-CSF-mobilized allografts and also phase I clinical studies. Both G-CSF and GM-CSF can be used to mobilize large numbers of blood stem cells which can be successfully used in the autograft setting not only providing trilineage engraftment but also accelerating recovery of platelets.

Strategies to improve the yield and long-term reconstituting capacity of blood stem cells

Two strategies using G-CSF and GM-CSF to mobilize blood stem cells are discussed above, i.e. cytokine alone and cytokine postchemotherapy. It seems that both approaches are effective. On the limited available published data, it would appear that a greater yield of blood stem cells can be obtained using colony-stimulating factors during recovery from chemotherapy, with the advantage that fewer leukaphereses may be required. The other advantage of this approach is that the blood stem cell harvest can thereby be scheduled during the initial chemotherapy program. The major disadvantage is that the timing of leukaphereses may be difficult and logistical problems may occur with the availability of resources. It may also not be appropriate to give further standard dose chemotherapy to a patient in remission and it is certainly not appropriate to give chemotherapy to a healthy allograft donor. It is probable that the marked mobilizing effect of certain kinds of chemotherapy is the consequence of reactive endogenous production of cytokine(s) as a response to myelosuppression. One obvious research goal will be to identify these growth factor(s) and to mimic the best cytokine combination for a reproducible, well-tolerated and optimal expansion/mobilization of the stem cell pool in the absence of prior chemotherapy.

There is evidence that the absolute number of blood stem cells infused (as measured by the surrogate assay for CFU-GM) is inversely correlated with the time to engraftment, although such a correlation has not been reported by all observers. The speed of hematopoietic recovery in an analysis of 74 patients by Gianni *et al.* (pers. comm.) was directly related to the number of CFU-GM infused, up to a value of 10^5 CFU-GM/kg, above which no further increase in the rate of recovery could be seen (Fig. 5.4). Time to neutrophil recovery was correlated ($r = 0.69$) with the logarithm of CFU-GM/kg infused. A similar result has been reported in a mouse model (Jones *et al.*, 1987). Strategies using other cytokines or combinations could possibly result in mobilization of different types of blood stem cells which could rapidly engraft without the need for large numbers.

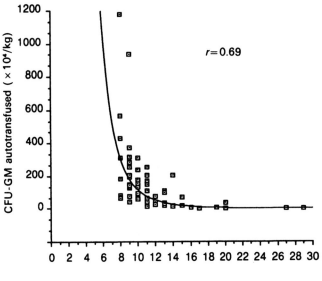

Fig. 5.4. Correlation between time to recovery and committed stem cell dose in 74 patients autografted with a combination of bone marrow and blood stem cells. Pre-transplant chemotherapy was either melphalan (200 mg/m²) or melphalan (120 mg/m²) plus 10–12.5 Gy fractionated total body irradiation.

Other colony-stimulating factors

Interleukin-3 (IL-3) has been shown to increase blood stem cells (Geissler *et al.*, 1989; Welniak *et al.*, 1991) including erythroid burst-forming units (BFU-E) and CFU-MK, although after chemotherapy the rise was several-fold less than that induced by GM-CSF (Siena *et al.*, 1991a). The sequential administration of IL-3 followed by GM-CSF after chemotherapy apparently results in an even greater increase in CFU-GM (Brugger *et al.*, 1991; A.M. Gianni *et al.*, personal communication). IL-3 is able to stimulate multiple lineages *in vitro* and there is evidence in a primate model (Winton *et al.*, 1990) that sequential IL-3 and GM-CSF results in preferential release of very early progenitors.

Phase I clinical trials of stem cell factor (SCF, kit ligand, steel factor) commenced in December 1991. *In vitro* it has synergistic activity with the various colony-stimulating factors resulting in large colony size and increased colony number (McNiece *et al.*, 1991; Cicuttini *et al.*, 1992). In baboons, SCF adminstration for 7–14 days has been shown to increase

CFU-GM in the marrow and also in peripheral blood (Andrews *et al.*, 1991). Similar effects on blood stem cells are seen in the peripheral blood of dogs given SCF (Schuening *et al.*, 1991).

There is growing evidence that IL-6 is involved in normal human megakaryopoiesis (Navarro *et al.*, 1991). IL-6 administration to mice (Hill *et al.*, 1991) and nonhuman primates (Mayer *et al.*, 1991) results in increased size and ploidy of megakaryocytes as well as increased platelet numbers in the peripheral blood. The use of IL-6 perhaps with G-CSF or GM-CSF may result in a relatively higher proportion of megakaryocyte progenitors released into the peripheral blood. The use of the combination of an 'early acting' factor (e.g. IL-1, IL-3, IL-6, SCF) with a 'late acting' factor (e.g. G-CSF, GM-CSF) may similarly result in greater numbers of circulating early progenitors and improve the clinical utility of this approach.

Conclusions and future directions

The application of hematopoietic growth factors for mobilization and collection of blood stem cells is likely to transform the field of blood stem cell transplants, at least for the nonmyeloid malignancies. Significant advantages in ease of use, improved scheduling, improved yields of stem cells, and accelerated engraftment potential all argue strongly for the incorporation of colony-stimulating factors into blood stem cell collection strategies. Determination of the optimum factor or combination of factors, dosage, scheduling, route of administration, and incorporation with chemotherapy regimens of various types awaits further study.

The use of colony-stimulating factors to mobilize blood stem cells has made allogeneic blood cell transplants a feasible proposition. For example, G-CSF could be safely administered to a normal allogeneic transplant donor for a period of 4–6 days allowing for collection of blood stem cells by leukapheresis. This has the potential of reducing morbidity for the donor by avoiding a general anesthetic and may provide benefit to the recipient in terms of more rapid engraftment. A successful sex-mismatched allograft of blood stem cells could be used to provide definitive evidence of the ability of blood stem cells to produce long-term engraftment in humans. If a single leukapheresis was sufficient and the percentage of CD34$^+$ cells could be used as a reliable surrogate for colony assays, blood stem cell allotransplants would be fairly straightforward procedures from the technical standpoint. A careful assessment of the risk of graft-versus-host disease would also need to be performed as a greater number of T cells would be infused with blood stem cells compared with bone marrow. It is probable that the number of infused T cells in a blood stem cell allotransplant will need to be controlled by using partial T cell depletion methods.

The use of hematopoietic growth factors to mobilize blood stem cells to support multiple courses of high dose (nonmyeloablative) chemotherapy in patients with solid tumors should be subjected to clinical trial. At present, none of the available colony-stimulating factors stimulate megakaryocytes *in vivo*, hence the use of blood stem cells is the only method currently available that will hasten platelet recovery after high doses of chemotherapy. Thus it seems likely that blood stem cells mobilized by hematopoietic growth factors will play an increasing role in the management of patients with hematologic and nonhematologic malignancies.

References

Andrews, R.G., Bertelmez, S.H., Knitter, G. *et al.* (1991). Recombinant human stem cell factor (SCF) stimulates increased numbers of peripheral blood and marrow CFU-GM, BFU-E, CFU-MIX, HPP-CFC, and CD34[+] cells in baboons. *Blood*, **78** (suppl. 1): 261a–no. 1036 (abstract).

Bolwell, B.J., Lichtin, A., Andresen, S. *et al.* (1991). G-CSF and peripheral primed progenitor cells (PPPC) enhances engraftment in autologous bone marrow transplantation (ABMT) for non-Hodgkin's lymphoma and Hodgkin's disease. *Blood*, **78**: 242a–no. 959 (abstract).

Brugger, W., Bross, K.J., Frisch, J., Schulz, G., Mertelsmann, R. & Kanz, L. (1991). Combined sequential administration of IL-3 + GM-CSF after polychemotherapy with etoposide, ifosfamide, and cisplatin. *Blood*, **78** (suppl. 1): 162a–no. 638 (abstract).

Cicuttini, F.M., Begley, C.G. & Boyd, A.W. (1992). The effect of recombinant stem cell factor (SCF) on purified CD-34-positive human umbilical cord blood progenitor cells. *Growth Factors*, **6**: 31–9.

Duhrsen, U., Villeval, J.L., Boyd, J., Kannourakis, G., Morstyn, G. & Metcalf, D. (1988). Effects of recombinant granulocyte colony-stimulating factor on hematopoietic progenitor cells in cancer patients. *Blood*, **72**: 2074–81.

Elias, A.D., Ayash, L., Anderson, K.C. *et al.* (1992a). Mobilization of peripheral blood progenitor cells (PBPC) by chemotherapy and GM-CSF for hematologic support after high-dose intensification for breast cancer. *Blood*, **79**: 3036–44.

Elias, A., Mazanet, R., Anderson, K. *et al.* (1992b). GM-CSF mobilized peripheral blood stem cell autografts: the DFCI/BIH experience. *Int. J. Cell Cloning*, **10** (suppl. 1): 149–51.

Geissler, K., Valent, P., Mayer, P. *et al.* (1989). RhIL-3 expands the pool of circulating hemopoietic stem cells in primates–synergism with RhGM-CSF. *Blood*, **74** (suppl. 1): 151a–no. 562 (abstract).

Gianni, A.M., Siena, S., Bregni, M., Tarella, C., Sciorelli, G.A. & Bonadonna, G. (1989a). Very rapid and complete haematopoietic reconstitution following myeloablative treatments: the role of circulating stem cells harvested after high-dose cyclophosphamide and GM-CSF. In *Autologous Bone Marrow Transplantation*, ed. K.A. Dicke, G. Spitzer, S. Jagannath & M.J.

Evinger-Hodges, 4th edn, pp. 723–31. The University of Texas Press, Houston.

Gianni, A.M., Siena, S., Bregni, M. *et al.* (1989b). Granulocyte-macrophage colony-stimulating factor to harvest circulating haemopoietic stem cells for autotransplantation. *Lancet*, **2**: 580–5.

Gianni, A.M., Siena, S., Bregni, M. *et al.* (1992). Granulocyte-macrophage colony-stimulating factor to harvest circulating haemopoietic stem cells for autotransplantation. In *Critical Papers in Bone Marrow Transplantation 1992 – An Anthology*, ed. R.L. Powles & E.C. Gordon-Smith (in press).

Gianni, A.M., Bregni, M., Siena, S. *et al.* (1993). Clinical usefulness and optimal harvesting of peripheral blood stem cells mobilized by high dose cyclophosphamide and rhGM-CSF. In *Peripheral Blood Stem Cell Autografts*, ed. P. Henon & E. Wunder. Springer-Verlag, Heidelberg (in press).

Groopman, J.E. (1988). Clinical applications of colony-stimulating factors. *Semin. Oncol.*, **15**: 27–33.

Haas, R., Ho, A.D., Bredthauer, U. *et al.* (1990). Successful autologous transplantation of blood stem cells mobilized with recombinant human granulocyte-macrophage colony-stimulating factor. *Exp Hematol*, **18**: 94–8.

Hill, R.J., Warren, M.K., Stenberg, P. *et al.* (1991). Stimulation of megakaryocyopoiesis in mice by human recombinant intereukin-6. *Blood*, **77**: 42–8.

Jones, R.J., Sharkis, S.J., Celano, P., Colvin, O.M., Rowley, S.D. & Sensenbrenner, L.L. (1987). Progenitor cell assays predict hematopoietic reconstitution after syngeneic transplantation in mice. *Blood*, **70**: 1186–92.

Juttner, C.A. & To, L.B. (1991). Peripheral blood stem cells: mobilization by myelosuppressive chemotherapy. In *Autologous Bone Marrow Transplantation*, ed. K.A. Dicke, J.O. Armitage, M.J. Dicke-Evinger. Proceedings of the Fifth International Symposium, Omaja, pp. 783–90. University of Nebraska Medical Center.

McNiece, I.K., Langley, K.E. & Zsebo, K.M. (1991). Recombinant human stem cell factor synergizes with GM-CSF, G-CSF, IL-3 and EPO to stimulate human progenitor cells of the myeloid and erythroid lineages. *Exp. Hematol.* **19**: 226–31.

Mayer, P., Geissler, K., Valent, P., Ceska, M., Bettelheim, P. & Liehl, E. (1991). Recombinant human interleukin 6 is a potent inducer of the acute phase response and elevates the blood platelets in nonhuman primates. *Exp. Hematol.*, **19**: 688–96.

Molineux, G., Pojda, Z., Hampson, I.N., Lord, B.I. & Dexter, T.M. (1990). Transplantation potential of peripheral blood stem cells induced by granulocyte colony-stimulating factor. *Blood*, **76**: 2153–8.

Navarro, S., Debili, N., Le Couedic, J.-P. *et al.* (1991). Interleukin-6 and its receptor are expressed by human megakaryocytes: in vitro effects on proliferation and endoreduplication. *Blood*, **77**: 461–71.

Pettengell, R., Demuynck, H., Testa, N.G. & Dexter, T.M. (1992). The engraftment capacity of peripheral blood stem cells (PBSC) mobilised with chemotherapy +/− G-CSF. *Int. J. Cell Cloning*, **10** (suppl. 1): 59–61.

Schuening, F.G., Storb, R., Appelbaum, F.R., Deeg, H.J. & Zsebo, K. (1991). Effect of recombinant canine stem cell factor (c-kit ligand) on hematopoiesis of normal dogs, after lethal total body irradiation without marrow transplant, and after DLA-identical littermate marrow transplants. *Blood*, **78** (suppl. 1): 23a–no. 82 (abstract).

Sheridan, W.P., Begley, C.G., Juttner, C.A. *et al.* (1992) Effect of peripheral-blood progenitor cells mobilised by filgrastim (G-CSF) on platelet recovery after high-dose chemotherapy. *Lancet*, **339**: 640–4.

Siena, S., Bregni, M., Brando, B., Ravagnani, F., Bonadonna, G. & Gianni, A.M. (1989). Circulation of $CD34^+$ hematopoietic stem cells in the peripheral blood of high-dose cyclophosphamide-treated patients: enhancements by intravenous recombinant human granulocyte-macrophage colony-stimulating factor. *Blood*, **74**: 1905–14.

Siena, S., Bregni, M., Di Nicola, M., Bonadonna, G. & Gianni, M. (1991a). Hematopoietic progenitor cells circulating in the peripheral blood of breast cancer patients treated with high dose cyclophosphamide (HD-CTX) and recombinant human interleukin-3 (rhIL-3). *Ann. Hematol.*, **20** (abstract).

Siena, S., Bregni, M., Brando, B. *et al* (1991b). Flow cytometry for clinical estimation of circulating hematopoietic progenitors for autologous transplantation in cancer patients. *Blood*, **77**: 138–47.

Socinski, M.A., Cannistra, S.A., Elias, A., Antman, K.H., Schnipper, L. & Griffin, J.D. (1988). Granulocyte-macrophage colony-stimulating factor expands the circulating haemopoietic progenitor cell compartment in man. *Lancet*, **1**: 1194–8.

To, L.B., Dyson, P.G., Branford, A. *et al.* (1987). Peripheral blood stem cells collected in very early remission produce rapid and sustained autologous hematopoietic reconstitution in acute non-lymphoblastic leukaemia. *Bone Marrow Transplant.*, **2**: 103–8.

Villeval, J.-L., Dührsen, U., Morstyn, G. & Metcalf, D. (1990). Effect of recombinant human granulocyte-macrophage colony stimulating factor on progenitor cells in patients with advanced malignancies. *Br. J. Haematol.*, **74**: 36–44.

Welniak, L.A., Alter, R., Jackson, J.D. *et al.* (1991). Interleukin-3 enhances collection of peripheral blood mononuclear cells and CFU-GM. *Blood*, **78** (suppl. 1): 224a–no. 885 (abstract).

Winton, E.F., Rozmiarek, S.K., Jacobs, P.C. *et al.* (1990). Marked increase in marrow and peripheral blood multi-lineage and megakaryocyte progenitor cells induced by short-course sequential recombinant human IL-3/GM-CSF in a non-human primate. *Blood*, **76**: (suppl. 1): 172a–1720.

6

Mobilizing and collecting blood stem cells

L.B. TO

Introduction

The technology of peripheral blood stem cell collection is a by-product of
the expertise in extracorporal blood component separation. By the early
1980s microprocessor-controlled, menu-driven automated blood cell
separators were capable of efficiently separating whole blood into
granulocytes, mononuclear cells, platelets and plasma in a closed continuous
flow system. Meanwhile it was shown that primitive hematopoietic stem
cells in peripheral blood coseparate with lymphocytes and monocytes on
density and centrifugal gradients and hematopoietic reconstitution could
be achieved with blood stem cells (Nothdurft et al., 1977; Fliedner et al.,
1979; Korbling et al., 1980; Abrams et al., 1981; Juttner et al., 1985). In
clinical studies, blood stem cell collections were most commonly performed
during recovery phase following myelosuppressive chemotherapy because
of the higher levels of hematopoietic stem cells during that time (Richman
et al., 1976; To et al., 1984) and the more rapid engraftment than when bone
marrow was used (Juttner et al., 1988; To et al., 1992b). Recent experiences
with hematopoietic growth factors and other cytokines show that they may
also enhance blood stem cell levels with or without myelosuppressive
chemotherapy (Gianni et al., 1989; Antman et al., 1990; Geissler et al.,
1990; Haas et al., 1989; Schaafsma et al., 1990; Fibbe et al., 1992; Sheridan
et al., 1992; Vose et al., 1992). Blood stem cells collected without
mobilization during steady phase hematopoiesis (Kessinger et al., 1986,
1988), during chronic phase of chronic myeloid leukemia (Goldman and
Lu, 1982) and from placenta at birth (cord blood) (Gluckman et al., 1989)
are other types of blood stem cell although their rate of engraftment is more
similar to that of bone marrow transplants. The technology of blood stem
cell collection and the different approaches to enhancing blood stem cell
levels are the two main issues addressed in this chapter.

Blood stem cell transplant experiences suggest strongly that peripheral blood cells contain both long-term marrow repopulating cells and committed progenitors. The former remain to be defined *in vitro* although several candidate phenotypes have been proposed (Sutherland *et al.*, 1990; Smith *et al.*, 1991; Baum *et al.*, 1992) while the latter can be measured as clonogenic colony-forming cells and by their expression of the CD34 antigen (Civin *et al.*, 1984). Several reports showed a significant correlation between hematopoietic reconstitutive capacity and the number of committed progenitors reinfused (Rowley *et al.*, 1991; Siena *et al.*, 1991; To *et al.*, 1990b, 1992b) so the term blood stem cell is used in a generic sense here to include both types of cell, although only committed progenitors are usually measured.

Blood stem cell collection

Machines

Hemonetics V30 was one of the first blood cell separators used. It and its successor V50 operated in an intermittent flow mode. The efficiency of blood stem cell collection has been improved by the lymphosurge procedure and more recently the counterflow centrifugation procedure (Schouten *et al.*, 1990), but both require major operator input.

Fenwal CS3000 and Cobe Spectra are the two most commonly used blood cell separators. They operate in a closed continuous flow mode and are generally easier to operate and produce less circulatory disturbance. The Spectra requires the operator to position the buffy coat but its product has minimal red cell and platelet contamination. The CS3000 is fully automated with two inbuilt procedures (1 and 3) suitable for blood stem cell apheresis. Its use in blood stem cell collection has been well described (To *et al.*, 1989) and the combined use of procedure 1 and a new small volume collection chamber has been shown to provide a comparable clean product (Bender, 1992) which would minimize prestorage processing and may have less clumping on thawing. Other continuous flow separators such as the Fresenius AS104 are still being evaluated.

Vascular access

Peripheral veins are the safest type of venous access for apheresis, although previous cytotoxic damage to veins, irradiation and recent surgery may dictate the use of other approaches such as subclavian silicon rubber catheters (Hickman's catheter). We prefer more rigid silastic catheters such as VASCATH so that patency is maintained even at high draw speed. The external jugular vein, the femoral vein and the inferior vena cava (via a translumbar catheter) (Haire *et al.*, 1989) are also alternatives.

Side-effects

Major side-effects are uncommon with continuous flow blood cell separators. Circulatory overload in pediatric subjects can be avoided by priming the extracorporal volume (Takaue *et al.*, 1989a; Lasky *et al.*, 1991). Citrate overdose and boredom can be relieved by a glass of calcium gluconate and friendly apheresis staff. Blockage of rigid subclavian catheters is uncommon in our institution, although one study reported 65% blockage with silicon rubber catheters (Haire *et al.*, 1990a). Flushing with heparinized saline or bolus injection of urokinase may relieve blockage. Urokinase infusion may be tried if the delay in apheresis is acceptable (Haire *et al.*, 1990b). Catheter sepsis usually requires catheter removal, besides the appropriate antibiotic and a short course of anticoagulant for septic thrombosis.

Blood product requirement varies among different mobilization protocols. During steady phase hematopoiesis both the hemoglobin levels and the platelet counts dropped following apheresis (Korbling *et al.*, 1980). In recovery phase collections the leukocyte and lymphocyte counts also decreased significantly (Haylock *et al.*, 1992a). Recent improvements in technology such as the Spectra and the use of procedure 1 and the small volume collection chamber on the CS3000 should reduce red cell and platelet depletion. Depletion is less of a problem with hematopoietic growth factor mobilization because myelosuppression does not occur.

Sustained cytopenia after blood stem cell collection was reported in two 3-year-old children with cancer, although blood counts normalized following high dose chemotherapy and blood stem cell rescue (Takaue *et al.*, 1989b). It was suggested that the blood stem cell is a major component of the hematopoietic cells in small children during hematopoietic recovery. This has not been reported following blood stem cell collections in adults, although we have observed transient leukopenia with leukocyte counts of $1.7 \times 10^9/l$ to $3.4 \times 10^9/l$ 2 weeks following granulocyte colony-stimulating factor (G-CSF) mobilization in three patients (L.B. To, unpublished data). Headache in patients with intracranial pathology had also been reported (Smith *et al.*, 1990).

Collection efficiency

Collection efficiency is the percentage of blood stem cells collected relative to the number of blood stem cells processed. The mononuclear cell and granulocyte/macrophage colony-forming unit (CFU-GM) collection efficiency of the CS3000 in published reports ranged from 55% to 75% (Lasky *et al.*, 1987; Haylock *et al.*, 1992a). We have recently reported a significant difference between the overall CFU-GM CE of 56% (based on the number of cells at start of apheresis and the blood volume processed) and the instantaneous collection efficiency of 95% (based on a comparison of the cells at the intake and the output line of the blood cell separator) (Haylock *et al.*, 1992a). The discrepancy was attributed to three nonmachine-related factors: (1) the fall in mononuclear cell and CFU-GM levels during apheresis, (2) dilution of blood by anticoagulant, and (3) the operational dead space in the blood cell separator at the start of apheresis. These data suggest that the current blood stem cell collection technology based on mononuclear cell collection is already quite optimal. The overall collection efficiency for the Spectra is similar to that of the CS3000 (Craig *et al.*, 1992), although no data on the instantaneous collection efficiency are available.

Future

The next generation of blood stem cell harvesters will probably be automated, closed, continuous flow systems with the additional capacity to capture stem cells specifically. Immunoabsorption, immunomagnetic beads or other solid phase systems are all candidates. Positive selection for $CD34^+$ cells will provide a much smaller volume of cells that reduces storage costs and possible side-effects, such as circulatory overload and dimethyl sulfoxide (DMSO) toxicity when reinfused. Such systems may also lead to depletion of tumor cells.

Determining the optimal time of blood stem cell collection

Assuming a CFU-GM target of 30×10^4/kg body weight in a 70 kg patient, a processed blood volume of 10 l, a PB CFU-GM level of 1×10^6/l during blood stem cell mobilization and a collection efficiency of 60%, two to three aphereses would provide sufficient stem cells. The levels of CFU-GM in hematopoietic growth factor mobilization are often higher (Siena *et al.*, 1989; Pettengell *et al.*, 1992), so as few as one apheresis may be sufficient. It then becomes important that aphereses are performed at the time of maximal blood stem cell levels. Various parameters to determine the optimal timing in recovery phase collections have been used: the leukocyte and platelet counts (To *et al.*, 1984; Gianni *et al.*, 1989), the rate of rise of the leukocyte count (Emminger *et al.*, 1990; To *et al.*, 1990c) and the level of CD34[+] cells measured by flow cytometry (Siena *et al.*, 1989; 1991). Of these, CD34[+] cell measurement is the most direct and the recently available fluorescein (FITC)-conjugated CD34 antibody, FITC-8G12, requires only 50 μl of heparinized whole blood, provides results on the same day and shows a significant correlation to the CFU-GM content (Siena *et al.*, 1991). Another directly conjugated CD34 antibody, FITC-QBEND10, used in the same assay, seems to provide less satisfactory resolution of positive cells (Ravagnani *et al.*, 1991). For units without access to a flow cytometer the APAAP technique is an alternative (To *et al.*, 1990a). Numerous reports have now confirmed that there is a close and significant correlation between the levels of CD34[+] cells and CFU-GM (Juttner *et al.*, 1990; Siena *et al.*, 1991; Bender *et al.*, 1992).

An additional advantage of CD34[+] cell measurements is that their level should provide an important index of both the early and the long-term hematopoietic reconstitutive capacity of blood stem cells. CD34[+] cells contain not only colony-forming cells that correlate with rapid engraftment (To *et al.*, 1986, 1992a; Reiffers *et al.*, 1988) but also more primitive cells as measured by the pre-progenitor or delta assay (Haylock *et al.*, 1992b) or as long-term culture initiating cells (LTC-IC) (Bender *et al.*, 1992; Pettengell *et al.*, 1992).

In recovery phase collections it is necessary to monitor blood stem cell levels and to coordinate apheresis and cryopreservation accordingly on a day-to-day basis. This is demanding on patients and the health unit alike. In comparison, hematopoietic growth factor mobilization may be simpler to administer. For instance, apheresis can be planned in G-CSF mobilization because the highest levels occurred between the fifth and seventh day of G-CSF administration (Sheridan *et al.*, 1992). The timings of collection in other HGF mobilization protocols are still under study.

Measures to enhance the levels of blood stem cells

Significance of high CFU-GM/CD34[+]

Faster neutrophil and platelet recovery, fewer febrile days, reduced blood product requirement and shorter hospitalizations following high dose therapy are some of the major advantages of blood stem cell rescue compared with bone marrow rescue. These advantages occurred with

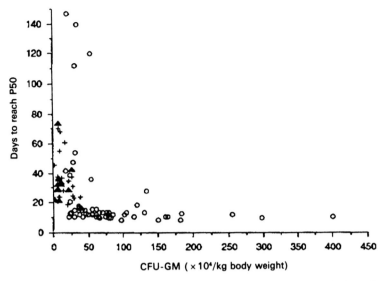

Fig. 6.1. Significant correlation between early platelet recovery and the colony-forming unit-granulocyte/macrophage (CFU-GM) dose given. P50 = number of days posttransplant to reach $50 \times ^9$ platelets/l. (O) Blood stem cell. (+) Allogeneic bone marrow transplant. (▲) Autologous bone marrow transplant.

blood stem cells collected during recovery phase from myelosuppressive chemotherapy or during hematopoietic growth factor administration or a combination of both (Juttner *et al.*, 1988; Antman *et al.*, 1990; Gianni *et al.*, 1990; Sheridan *et al.*, 1992; To *et al.*, 1992b) but not with blood stem cells collected during steady phase hematopoiesis (Kessinger *et al.*, 1988). This difference between mobilized and steady phase blood stem cell probably results from the difference in the number of stem cells. A threshold of 15 to 50×10^4 CFU-GM/kg body weight below which rapid engraftment may not occur has been suggested by various laboratories (To *et al.*, 1986, 1990b, 1992b; Juttner *et al.*, 1987; Reiffers *et al.*, 1988). Figures 6.1 and 6.2 show the regression analysis of early platelet and neutrophil recovery and the CFU-GM dose in 65 patients transplanted in a single institution (To *et al.*, 1992b). They demonstrate both the significant correlation with the CFU-GM dose and the presence of a threshold of 30×10^4 to 50×10^4 CFU-GM/kg body weight.

CD34 and CFU-GM

There is an increasing trend to define the blood stem cell apheresis target on the basis of CD34$^+$ cells instead of CFU-GM. CD34 results are available

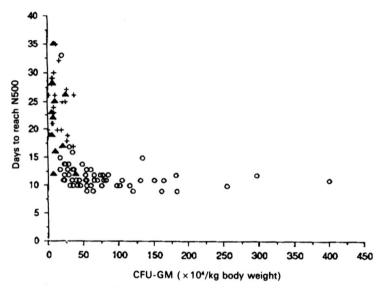

Fig. 6.2. Significant correlation between early neutrophil recovery and the colony-forming unit-granulocyte/macrophage CFU-GM dose given. N500 = number of days posttransplant to reach 0.5×10^9 neutrophils/l. (O) Blood stem cell. (+) Allogeneic bone narrow transplant. (▲) Autogenous bone marrow transplant.

faster and have less variability between laboratories than the assay system for CFU-GM. Berenson *et al.* (1991) suggested 1×10^6 CD34[+] cells/kg body weight using bone marrow-derived cells, whereas Sienna *et al.* (1991) suggested 7.8×10^6/kg body weight using GM-CSF and cyclophosphamide-mobilized blood stem cells.

Other factors affecting engraftment

Other factors in mobilized peripheral blood may also contribute to the rapid hematopoietic reconstitution. Recovery phase blood stem cells containing low numbers of CFU-GM enhanced the rate of hematopoietic reconstitution when given together with bone marrow cells (Bell *et al.*, 1987; Lopez *et al.*, 1991; Sheridan *et al.*, 1992), whereas steady phase blood stem cells did not (Lobo *et al.*, 1991; Nademanee *et al.*, 1992). These findings suggest that cytokines and accessory cells may be partly responsible.

Blood stem cells collected during chronic phase of CML are an exception to the observation that unmobilized blood stem cells do not produce rapid engraftment. They are different from other steady phase collections because of the higher number of CFU-GM and their neoplastic origin.

Blood stem cell mobilization protocols
Recovery phase following myelosuppressive chemotherapy

This type of mobilization protocol has been well described since the mid-1980s. Increased levels of stem cells and LTC-IC were often present when the leukocyte and platelet counts were rapidly rising during hematopoietic recovery following cytotoxic-induced myelosuppression (Richman *et al.*, 1976; To *et al.*, 1984; Bender *et al.*, 1992). Both single high doses of cyclophosphamide (4–7 gm/m²) and different combination chemotherapy regimens have been used. The common factor seems to be sufficient myelosuppression to cause more than a few days of cytopenia. The advantage of this approach is that blood stem cell mobilization occurs during effective anti-tumor treatment so that no additional mobilization therapy is necessary. The disadvantages are the associated cytopenic risks and the logistic requirement for close monitoring of the recovery phase to perform apheresis at the optimal time. Heavily pretreated patients may show little or no mobilization.

Laporte *et al.* (1990) reported that folinic acid, given to patients with acute myeloid leukaemia who were undergoing induction or consolidation chemotherapy, enhanced the increase seen during recovery phase. It is not clear whether this enhancing effect occurs in other diseases.

Hematopoietic growth factors and other cytokines

G-CSF Duhrsen *et al.* (1988) showed that following continuous intravenous infusion of G-CSF myeloid, erythroid and multilineage progenitors rose in the blood after 5–7 days, an effect not explicable by known *in vitro* activities of G-CSF. In a subsequent study Sheridan *et al.* (1992) showed that G-CSF administration led to a median 63-fold increase in the CFU-GM collected by apheresis, although little or no increase in progenitors occurred in some heavily pretreated patients. G-CSF mobilized blood stem cells, when given with bone marrow and G-CSF postgraft, produced more rapid platelet engraftment than that seen after bone marrow alone or bone marrow plus G-CSF postgraft. The same rapid and sustained engraftment occurred in patients transplanted with G-CSF mobilized blood stem cells without bone marrow (W. Sheridan, unpublished data).

GM-CSF Socinski *et al.* (1988) reported an 18-fold increase in peripheral blood CFU-GM after 3–7 days of GM-CSF at 4–64 μg/kg per day as a continuous intravenous infusion. Haas *et al.* (1990) reported a mean

8.5-fold increase in peripheral blood CFU-GM after 10 days (median) in 11 patients with lymphoma or sarcoma receiving GM-CSF at 250 μg per day as a continuous intravenous infusion. Six patients were transplanted with GM-CSF mobilized blood stem cells with a median mononucleated cell dose of 5.0×10^9 per patient and a median CFU-GM dose of 28.6×10^4 per patient. One patient who had progressive bone marrow disease posttransplant did not show engraftment. In the other five patients the median time to reach 0.5×10^9/l neutrophils and a stable platelet count of $> 20 \times 10^9$/lwas 28.5 and 39 days, respectively. Such an engraftment rate was no different from that in bone marrow transplantation but it is noteworthy that the CFU-GM dose was well below 1×10^4/kg body weight.

IL-3 In rhesus monkeys, Geissler *et al.* (1990) reported a 12–13-fold increase in peripheral blood progenitors after 11–14 days of IL-3 at 33 μg/kg per day subcutaneously. In human, Vose *et al.* (1992) reported a 12-fold increase in peripheral blood CFU-GM in patients with Hodgkin's disease after 11 days (mean) of IL-3 at 125 μg/kg per day intravenously.

IL-3/GM-CSF In rhesus monkeys, Geissler *et al.* (1990) compared IL-3 (33 μg/kg per day subcutaneously for 11–14 days) followed by GM-CSF (5.5 μg/kg per day for 5–14 days) with either GM-CSF or IL-3 alone. There was a 63-fold increase in peripheral blood CFU-GM in the sequential protocol compared with 12- and 14-fold, respectively, in the others. No published data is available in humans or with the GM-CSF/IL-3 fusion protein PIXY 321 (Williams & Park, 1991).

Stem cell factor (SCF) In baboons, Andrews *et al.* (1991) described a 10–1000-fold increase in CFU-GM and BFU-E as well as detectable levels of CFU-Mix and HPP-CFU in blood after 200 μg/kg per day of stem cell factor given either subcutaneously or intravenously.

Other cytokines Schaafsma *et al.* (1990) described a 20-fold increase in peripheral blood stem cells 5 days after cessation of 5 days of IL-2 at 3×10^6 μg/m² per day. Fibbe *et al.* (1992) described a 30-fold increase in CFU-GM and a 10-fold increase in $CFU-S_{12}$ in peripheral blood of Balb/C mice 4–8 h after 1 μg of IL-1 and these peripheral blood cells had long-term hematopoietic reconstitutive capacity. Because of the known toxicity profile of IL-1, it is not clear whether this will be testable in humans.

It thus seems that quite a number of cytokines are capable of enhancing the level of blood stem cells. No cytopenia occurs and the subcutaneous route is probably just as effective in most cases so mobilization could be performed on an outpatient basis. G-CSF is currently the best-defined protocol while cytokines acting on primitive progenitors such as SCF and IL-3 are still being studied.

Hematopoietic growth factors following myelosuppressive chemotherapy

The Milan group reported higher yields of CFU-GM $(26-29 \times 10^6/$ apheresis) in patients receiving cyclophosphamide 7 gm/m^2 on day 0 and GM-CSF at 5.5 μg/kg body weight as a continuous intravenous infusion from day 1 or day 5 to day 14 than in patients who received cyclophosphamide alone $(3.3 \times 10^6$ per apheresis). Patients who received GM-CSF from day 1 to day 7 or day 10 had intermediate yields $(10 \times 10^6$ per apheresis) (Tarella *et al.*, 1991). Patients receiving GM-CSF also experienced more rapid neutrophil and platelet recovery (Gianni *et al.*, 1990). The Boston group reported that GM-CSF at 5 μg/kg twice daily subcutaneously enhanced CFU-GM yield during recovery phase collection following AFM (adriamycin, 5-fluorouracil and methotrexate) induction chemotherapy in breast cancer patients (Antman *et al.*, 1990).

Similarly, G-CSF at 230 μg/m^2 daily subcutaneously given following doxorubicin 35 mg/m^2 intravenously day 1 and etoposide 100 mg/m^2 orally days 1–5 increased the peripheral blood CFU-GM, BFU-E and CFU-Mix 59-fold compared with pretreatment levels. The peak increase occurred between day 7 and day 9 of G-CSF administration. In chemotherapy cycles without G-CSF the increase was only 13-fold (Pettengell *et al.*, 1992).

Brugger *et al.* (1992) reported that the fold-increase in peripheral blood stem cells following chemotherapy-induced myelosuppression in patients given sequential IL-3 (250 μg/m^2 subcutaneously on days 1–5) and GM-CSF (250 μg/m^2 subcutaneously on days 6–15) was double that seen in patients given GM-CSF alone (days 1–15) compared with those who received chemotherapy but no cytokines. The number of CD34$^+$ cells was not different between the HGF groups. The authors postulated that there were both primitive and committed stem cells in the CD34$^+$ cells based on the presence of CD34$^+$/CD33$^-$, CD34$^+$/CD38$^-$ and CD34$^+$/HLA-DR$^-$ cells.

Other factors affecting mobilization

Besides the mobilization stimulus, there are other factors that affect the number of blood stem cells collected. In recovery phase blood stem cell collection, the severity of myelosuppression bears an inverse relation to the level of CFU-GM (To *et al.*, 1992a). Another factor that appears important

Table 6.1. *Summary of blood stem cell mobilization protocols*

Stimulus	Timing of mobilization	Fold-increase in BSC	Fold-increase in WCC	Bone marrow cellularity	Bone marrow stem cells (%)
Exercise, ACTH, endotoxin	3–5h	2–4	Increased	ND	ND
Dextran sulfate	3–5h	4–8	4	ND	ND
IL-1 (mouse)	4–8h	10–30	5	NC / Increased 48 h	NC / Increased 48 h
G-CSF	5–8 days	0–100	5–10	Increased	Decreased
GM-CSF	5–11 days	10–18[a]	2–5	Normal/increased	Decreased
IL-3	11 days	2–12[a]	Normal/increased	Normal/increased	Normal
IL-3+GM-CSF (baboons)	14–18 days	60[b]	2	Normal/increased	Normal
SCF (baboons)	7–14 days	10–600	4	2	Normal
Cyclophosphamide	14–20 days	0–100	Recovery from myelosuppression	Decreased/normal	Increased
Chemotherapy + G-CSF	12–14 days	3–300	Normal/increased	ND	ND
Chemotherapy + GM-CSF	15–19 days	8 × chemotherapy	Normal/increased	ND	ND
Chemotherapy + IL-3 + GM-CSF	15–19 days	2 × chemotherapy +GM-CSF	Normal/increased	ND	ND

ACTH, adrenocorticotrophic hormone; BSC, blood stem cell; CSF, colony-stimulating factor; G, granulocyte; GM, granulocyte/macrophage; IL, interleukin; SCF, stem cell factor; NC, no change; ND, not done/not known; WCC, white cell count.
[a] No data on the lower limit of range quoted.
[b] Mean fold increase.

in both chemotherapy or hematopoietic growth factor mobilizations is the amount of previous chemotherapy and indirectly the hematopoietic reserve. Heavily pretreated patients generally responded less satisfactorily in recovery phase (To *et al.*, 1990b), G-CSF (Sheridan *et al.*, 1992) or GM-CSF (Haas *et al.*, 1990) or combined hematopoietic growth factor (HGF)-chemotherapy mobilizations (Brugger *et al.*, 1992). It is noteworthy that HGF that acts directly or synergistically on primitive hematopoietic cells, e.g. SCF or HGF combinations that may be more effective in blood stem cell mobilization in heavily pretreated patients are still under study.

Other mobilization protocols

Early studies showed that exercise, adrenocorticotropic hormone and endotoxin caused a two to four fold increase in peripheral blood CFU-GM (Cline and Golde, 1977; Barrett *et al.*, 1978). Dextran sulfate was first used in dogs to mobilize blood stem cells but human studies have not been performed until recently because of possible toxicities such as anaphylaxis, liver damage and bleeding tendency. Ma *et al.* (1992) showed that in normal subjects dextran sulfate (MW 35000) at 15–20 mg/kg intravenously produced a four to eight-fold increase in CFU-GM in 3–5 h without significant toxicity. The increases appeared to be transient, however, and the clinical utility of such approaches is yet to be defined.

Mechanisms of blood stem cell mobilization

The wide varieties of mobilization stimulus illustrate that multiple pathways may be involved. Mobilization may occur within hours or may take up to 3 weeks. Release is likely to be the predominant factor in the former, while proliferation may also be involved in the latter (Table 6.1). In IL-3 and SCF mobilization the bone marrow stem cell levels remain unchanged while in GM-CSF and G-CSF mobilizations they often decrease in incidence. Recovery phase protocols require a period of cytopenia while hematopoietic growth factor mobilization does not. The efficacy of G-CSF cannot be explained by its known *in vitro* activity on granulocytic progenitors and the effect of IL-1 further proves that mobilization may occur via indirect pathways. In protocols associated with proliferation of bone marrow, it is still necessary to explain the egress of large numbers of stem cells into the blood.

There is now increasing evidence in murine and human systems that primitive hematopoietic cells, including LTC–IC, specifically bind to as yet unidentified components of the bone marrow stroma (Verfaille *et al.*, 1990;

Gordon, 1990). This possibly explains why primitive hematopoietic cells do not usually circulate in peripheral blood. A large number of adhesion receptors have been identified on hematopoietic cells (Arkin *et al.*, 1990; Lewinsohn *et al.*, 1990; Liesveld *et al.*, 1991; Simmons *et al.*, 1992) and some of their ligands have been demonstrated on bone marrow stroma (Simmons *et al.*, 1992; Spooncer *et al.*, 1983). Thus hematopoietic cell–stromal cell interactions mediated by these molecules are likely to represent a major component of the mechanisms that retain hematopoietic stem cells within the bone marrow under steady state conditions. Conversely, a modulation of these interactions may be the final common pathway for different mobilization protocols and may provide the basis for new mobilization strategies.

It is possible that cytokines also play a central role in alterations of the hematopoietic cell–stromal cell interaction. Cells comprising the bone marrow stroma have been shown to produce a wide variety of cytokines (Clark & Kamen, 1987). These cytokines may contribute to the physiological retention of primitive cells within the bone marrow by regulating the expression and function of adhesion receptors and their ligands on stem and stromal cells or by mediating stem–stromal cell adhesion directly via binding of cytokine receptors expressed by the stem cells with cytokines present either as integral membrane proteins on stromal cells or bound to their extracellular matrix (Clark & Kamen, 1987; Roberts *et al.*, 1988). The paradigm for this latter type of interaction is illustrated by the product of the c-*kit* proto oncogene that functions as a cell surface receptor for SCF expressed as an integral membrane protein by stromal cells (Flanagan *et al.*, 1991). Such hypotheses may explain the efficacy of different cytokines in mobilization. Even recovery phase mobilization may be cytokine mediated as postchemotherapy recovery is probably cytokine driven. We have found that $CD34^+$ cells from cyclophosphamide mobilization have a lower incidence of c-*kit* gene product expression (mean $18(\pm 8)\%$, $n=4$) compared with those from steady phase bone marrow (mean $77(\pm 12)$ $n=8$) (Ashman *et al.*, 1991). The intensity of expression of the c-*kit* gene product is also lower. Cyclophosphamide-mobilized $CD34^+$ cells also tend to be rhodamine 123^{dull} and in G_0. Functional tests of adherence are in process to assess the significance of these findings.

Conclusion

There is little doubt that mobilized blood stem cells make high dose tumoricidal therapy safer because of rapid engraftment. Whether the wider application of high dose therapy leads to better quality of life and tumor control in more patients is still under study. The increasing understanding of blood stem cell mobilization nonetheless enables collection of sufficient blood stem cells in most patients eligible for high dose therapy so that myelotoxicity is becoming less and less a dose limiting factor. Safer dosage escalation would make it easier to study the question of tumor control. Hematopoietic growth factors are already making mobilization safer and more effective and modulation of the interaction between hematopoietic stroma and stem cells may provide another strategy to enhance mobilization. Stem cell selection technology may provide cleaner blood stem cells for transplant, although its most promising application may be in making available large numbers of primitive hematopoietic cells at high purity for further genetic and cellular modifications. Mobilized blood stem cells may contain a much higher percentage of CD34$^+$ cells than steady phase bone marrow, therefore they would be particularly suitable for CD34 selection.

References

Abrams, R.A., McCormack, K., Bowles, C. & Deisseroth, A.B. (1981). Cyclophosphamide treatment expands the circulating hematopoietic stem cell pool in dogs. *J. Clin. Invest.*, **67**: 1392–9.

Andrews, R.G., Knitter, G.H., Bartelmez, S.H. *et al.* (1991). Recombinant human stem cell factor, a c-*kit* ligand, stimulates hematopoiesis in primate. *Blood*, **78**: 1975–80.

Antman, K., Elias, A., Hunt, M. *et al.* (1990). GM-CSF potentiated peripheral blood progenitor (PBPC) collection and use after high dose chemotherapy. *Blood*, **76** (suppl. 1): 526a (abstract).

Arkin, I.S., Naprstek, B., Guarini, L., Ferronr, S. & Lipton, J.M. (1990). Expression of intercellular adhesion molecule-1 (CD54) on hemapoietic progenitors. *Blood*, **77**: 948–53.

Ashman, L.K., Cambareri, A.C., To, L.B., Levinsky, R.J. & Juttner, C.A. (1991). Expression of the YB5.B8 antigen (*c-kit* proto-oncogene product) in normal human bone marrow. *Blood*, **78**: 30–37.

Barrett, A.J., Longhurst, P., Sneath, P. & Watson, J.M. (1978). Mobilization of CFU-C by exercise and ACTH induced stress in man. *Exp. Hematol.*, **6**: 590–4.

Baum, C.M., Weissman, I.L., Tsukamoto, A.S., Buckle, A.M. & Peault, A.B. (1992). Isolation of a candidate human hematopoietic stem-cell population. *Proc. Natl. Acad. Sci. USA*, **89**: 2804–8.

Bell, A.J., Oscier, D.G., Figes, A. & Hamblin, T.J. (1987). Use of circulating stem cells to accelerate myeloid recovery after autologous bone marrow transplantation. *Br. J. Haematol.*, **67**: 252–3.

Bender, J.G. (1992). Harvesting of peripheral blood stem cells with the Fenwal CS3000 Plus Cell Separator and a small volume collection chamber. *Int. J. Cell Cloning*, **10**: 79–82.

Bender, J.G., Unverzagt, K.L., Walker, D.E. *et al.* (1992). Characterization of CD34$^+$ cells mobilized to the peripheral blood during the recovery from cyclophosphamide chemotherapy. *Int. J. Cell Cloning*, **10**: 23–6.

Berenson, R.J., Bensinger, W.I., Hill, R.S. *et al.* (1991). Engraftment after infusion of CD34$^+$ marrow cells in patients with breast cancer or neuroblastoma. *Blood*, **77**: 1717–22.

70	*L.B. To*

Brugger, W., Bross, K., Frisch, J. *et al.* (1992). Mobilization of peripheral blood progenitor cells by sequential administration of interleukin-3 and granulocyte-macrophage colony-stimulating factor following polychemotherapy with etoposide, ifosfamide and cisplatin. *Blood*, **79**: 1193–200.

Civin, C.I., Strauss, L.C., Brovall, C., Fackler, M.J., Schwartz, J.F. & Shaper, J.H. (1984). Antigenic analysis of hematopoiesis. III. A hematopoietic progenitor cell surface antigen defined by a monoclonal antibody raised against KG-1a cells. *J. Immunol.*, **133**: 157–65.

Cline, M.J. & Golde, D.W. (1977). Mobilization of hematopoietic stem cells (CFU-C) into the peripheral blood of man by endotoxin. *Exp. Hematol.*, **5**: 186–90.

Clark, S.C. & Kamen, R. (1987). The human hematopoietic colony-stimulating factors. *Science*, **236**: 1229–37.

Craig, J.I.O., Anthony, R.S., Smith, S.M. *et al.* (1992). Comparison of the Cobe Spectra and Baxter CS3000 cell separators for the collection of peripheral blood stem cells from patients with hematological malignancies. *Int. J. Cell Cloning*, **10**: 82–5.

Duhrsen, U., Villeval, J.L., Boyd, J., Kannourakis, G., Morstyn, G. & Metcalf, D. (1988). Effects of recombinant human granulocyte-colony stimulating factor on haemopoietic progenitor cells in cancer patients. *Blood*, **72**: 2074–81.

Emminger, W., Emminger-Schmidmeier, W., Hocker, P., Gerhartl, C., Kundi, M. & Gadner, H. (1990). The median daily increment of leukocytes during hematopoietic recovery reflects the myeloid progenitor cell yield during leukapheresis in children. *Bone Marrow Transplant.*, **5**: 419–24.

Fibbe, W.E., Hamilton, M.S., Laterveer, L.L. *et al.* (1992). Sustained engraftment of mice transplanted with IL-1 primed blood-derived stem cells. *J. Immunol.*, **148**: 417–21.

Flanagan, J.G., Chan, D.C. & Leder, P. (1991). Transmembrane form of the kit ligand growth factor is determined by alternative splicing and is missing in the Sld mutant. *Cell*, **64**: 1025–35.

Fliedner, T.M., Korbling, M., Arnold R. *et al.* (1979). Collection and cryopreservation of mononuclear blood leukocytes and of CFU-C in man. *Exp. Hematol.*, **7** (suppl. 5): 398–408.

Geissler, K., Valent, P., Mayer, P. *et al.* (1990). Recombinant human interleukin-3 expands the pool of circulating hematopoietic progenitor cells in primates and synergism with recombinant granulocyte/macrophage colony-stimulating factor. *Blood*, **75**: 2305–10.

Gianni, A.M., Bregni, M., Siena, S. *et al.* (1990). Recombinant human granulocyte-macrophage colony-stimulating factor reduces hematologic toxicity and widens clinical applicability of high-dose cyclophosphamide treatment in breast cancer and non-Hodgkin's lymphoma. *J. Clin. Oncol.*, **8**: 768–78.

Gianni, A.M., Siena, S., Bregni, M. *et al.* (1989). Granulocyte-macrophage colony-stimulating factor to harvest circulating haemopoietic stem cells for autotransplantation. *Lancet*, **2**: 580–5.

Gluckman, E., Broxmeyer, H.E., Auerback, A.D. *et al.* (1989). Hematopoietic reconstitution in a patient with Fanconi's anemia by means of umbilical-cord blood from an HLA-identical sibling. *N. Engl. J. Med.*, **321**: 1174–8.

Goldman, J.M. & Lu, D.P. (1982). New approaches in chronic granulocytic leukemia –origin, prognosis, and treatment. *Semin. Hematol.*, **19**: 241–56.

Gordon, M.Y. (1990). Haemapoietic progenitor cell binding to the environment *in vitro. Exp. Hematol.*, **18**: 837–42.

Haas, R., Ho, A.D., Bredthauer, U. *et al.* (1990). Successful autologous transplantation of blood stem cells mobilized with recombinant human granulocyte-macrophage colony-stimulating factors. *Exp. Hematol.*, **18**: 94–8.

Haire, W.D., Edney, J.A., Landmark, J.D. & Kessinger, A. (1990a). Thrombotic complications of subclavian apheresis catheters in cancer patients: prevention with heparin infusion. *J. Clin. Apheresis*, **5**: 188–91.

Haire, W.D., Lieberman, R.P., Lund, G.B. & Edney, J. (1990b). Obstructed central venous catheters. *Cancer*, **66**: 2279–85.

Haire, W.D., Lieberman, R.P., Lund, G.B., Wieczorek, B.M., Armitage, J.O. & Kessinger, A. (1989). Translumbar inferior vena cava catheters: safty and efficacy in peripheral blood stem cell transplantation. *Transfusion*, **30**: 511–15.

Haylock, D.N., Canty, A., Thorp, D., Dyson, P.G., Juttner, C.A. & To, L.B. (1992a). A discrepancy between the instantaneous and the overall collection efficiency of the Fenwal CS3000 for peripheral blood stem cell apheresis. *J. Clin. Apheresis*, **7**: 6–11.

Haylock, D.N., To, L.B., Dowse, T.L., Juttner, C.A. & Simmons, P.J. (1992b). Ex vivo expansion and maturation of peripheral blood CD34$^+$ cells into the myeloid lineage. *Blood*, **80**: 1405–12.

Juttner, C.A., To, L.B., Haylock, D.N., Branford, A. & Kimber, R.J. (1985). Circulating autologous stem cells collected from acute non-lymphoblastic leukaemia produce prompt but incomplete haemopoietic reconstitution after high dose melphalan or supralethal chemoradiotherapy. *Br. J. Haematol.*, **61**: 739–46.

Juttner, C.A., To. L.B., Ho, J.Q.K., Thorp, D.L. & Kimber, R.J. (1987). Successful peripheral blood stem-cell autograft with a near critical dose of myeloid progenitor cells in acute non-lymphoblastic leukaemia in relapse. *Med. J. Aust.*, **147**: 292–3.

Juttner, C.A., To, L.B., Ho, J.Q.K. *et al.* (1988). Early lympho-hemopoietic recovery after autografting using peripheral blood stem cells in acute non-lymphoblastic leukemia. *Transplant. Proc.*, **20**: 40–3.

Juttner, C.A., To, L.B., Haylock, D.N. *et al.* (1990). Approaches to blood stem cell mobilisation. Initial Australian clinical results. *Bone Marrow Transplant.*, **5** (suppl. 1): 22–4.

Kessinger, A., Armitage, J.O., Landmark, J.D., Smith, D.M. & Weisenburger, D.D. (1988). Autologous peripheral hematopoietic stem cell transplantation restores hematopoietic function following marrow ablative therapy. *Blood*, **71**: 723–7.

Kessinger, A., Armitage, J.O., Landmark, J.D. & Weisenberger, D.D. (1986). Reconstitution of hematopoietic function with autologous cryopreserved circulating stem cells. *Exp. Hematol.*, **14**: 192–6.

Korbling, M., Fliedner, T.M. & Pflieger, H. (1980). Collection of large quantities of granulocyte/macrophage progenitor cells (CFUs) in man by continuous-flow leukapheresis. *Scand. J. Haematol.*, **24**: 22–8.

Laporte, J.P., Douay, L., Allieri, A. *et al.* (1990). Expansion by folinic acid of the peripheral blood progenitor pool after chemotherapy: its use in autografting in acute leukaemia. *Br. J. Haematol.*, **74**: 445–51.

Lasky, L.C., Fox, S.B., Smith, J. & Bostrom, B. (1991). Collection and use of peripheral blood stem cells in very small children. *Bone Marrow Transplant.*, **7**: 281–4.

Lasky, L.C., Smith, J.A., McCullough, J. & Zanjani, E.D. (1987). Three-hour collection of committed and multipotent hematopoietic progenitor cells by apheresis. *Transfusion*, **27**: 276–8.

Lewinsohn, D.M., Nagler, A., Ginzton, N., Greenberg, P. & Butcher, E.C. (1990). Hematopoietic progenitor cell expression of the H-CAM (CD44) homing-associated adhesion molecule. *Blood*, **75**: 589–95.

Liesveld, J.L., Winslow, J.M., Kempski, M.C., Ryan, D.H., Brennan, J.K. & Abboud, C.N. (1991). Adhesive interactions of normal and leukemic human CD34⁺ myeloid progenitors: role of marrow stromal, fibroblast, and cytomatrix components. *Exp. Hematol.*, **19**: 63–70.

Lobo, F., Kessinger, A., Landmark, J.D. *et al.* (1991). Addition of peripheral blood stem cells collected without mobilization techniques to transplanted autologous bone marrow did not hasten marrow recovery following myeloablative therapy. *Bone Marrow Transplant.*, **8**: 389–392.

Lopez, M., Mortel, O., Pouillart, P. *et al.* (1991). Acceleration of hemopoietic recovery after autologous bone marrow transplantation by low doses of peripheral blood stem cells. *Bone Marrow Transplant.*, **7**: 173–81.

Ma, E.P., Guo, S.H., Wei, H.D. *et al.* (1992). Experimental study and normal individual trial of hemopoietic stem cell mobilizer DS. *Int. J. Cell Cloning*, **10**: 41–4.

Nademanee, A., Schmidt, G.M., Sniecinski, I., Dagis, A.C. & Forman, S.J. (1992). High-dose therapy followed by autologous bone marrow transplantation with or without peripheral stem cells in patients with lymphoid malignancies. *Int. J. Cell Cloning*, **10**: 165–7.

Nothdurft, W., Bruch, C., Fliedner, T.M. & Ruber, E. (1977). Studies on the regeneration of the CFUc-population in blood and bone marrow of lethally irradiated dogs after autologous transfusion of cryopreserved mononuclear blood cells. *Scand. J. Haematol.*, **19**: 470–81.

Pettengell, R., Demuynck, H., Testa, N.G. & Dexter, T.M. (1992). The engraftment capacity of peripheral blood progenitor cells (PBPC) mobilized with chemotherapy +/− G-CSF. *Int. J. Cell Cloning*, **10**: 59–61.

Ravagnani, F., Siena, S., Bregni, M. *et al.* (1991). Methodologies to estimate circulating hematopoietic progenitors for autologous transplantation in cancer patients. *Haematologica (Pavia)*, **76** (suppl. 1): 46–9.

Reiffers, J., Leverger, G., Marit, G. *et al.* (1988). Hematopoietic reconstitution after autologous blood stem cell transplantation. *Bone Marrow Transplantation: Current Controversies. Proceedings of Sandoz-UCLA Symposium*, ed. R.P. Gale & R.E. Champlin, p. 313. Alan R. Liss, New York.

Richman, C.M., Weiner, R.S. & Yankee, R.A. (1976). Increase in circulating stem cells following chemotherapy in man. *Blood*, **47**: 1031–9.

Roberts, R., Gallagher, J., Spooner, E., Allen, T.D., Bloomfield, F. & Dexter, T.M. (1988). Heparan sulphate bound growth factors: a mechanism for stromal cell mediated haemopoiesis. *Nature*, **332**: 376–8.

Rowley, S.D., Piantadosi, S., Marcellus, D.C. *et al.* (1991). Analysis of factors predicting speed of hematologic recovery after transplantation with 4-hydroperoxycyclophosphamide-purged autologous bone marrow grafts. *Bone Marrow Transplant.*, **7**: 183–92.

Schaafsma, M.R., Fibbe, W.E., van Der Harst, D. *et al.* (1990). Increased numbers of circulating haematopoietic progenitor cells after treatment with high-dose interleukin-2 in cancer patients. *Br. J. Haematol.*, **76**: 180–5.

Schouten, H.C., Kessinger, A., Smith, D.M. *et al.* (1990). Counterflow centrifugation apheresis for the collection of autologous peripheral blood stem cells from patients with malignancies. *J. Clin. Apheresis*, **5**: 140–4.

Sheridan, W.P., Begley, C.G., Juttner, C.A. *et al.* (1992). Effect of peripheral-blood progenitor cells mobilized by filgrastim (G-CSF) on platelet recovery after high-dose chemotherapy. *Lancet*, **339**: 640–4.

Siena, S., Bregni, M., Brando, B. *et al.* (1991). Flow cytometry for clinical estimation of circulating hematopoietic progenitors for autologous transplantation in cancer patients. *Blood*, **77**: 400–9.

Siena, S., Bregni, M., Brando, B., Ravagnani, F., Bonadonna, G. & Gianni, A.M. (1989). Circulation of $CD34^+$ hematopoietic stem cells in the peripheral blood of high-dose cyclophosphamide-treated patients: enhancement by intravenous recombinant human granulocyte-macrophage colony-stimulating factor. *Blood*, **74**: 1905–14.

Simmons, P.J., Mazinovsky, B., Lonenecker, B.M., Berenson, R., Torok-Storb, B. & Gallatin, W.M. (1992). VCAM-1 expressed by bone marrow stromal cells mediates the binding of haemopoietic progenitor cells. *Blood*, **80**: 388–95.

Smith, C., Gasparetto, C., Collins, N. *et al.* (1991). Purification and partial characterization of a human hematopoietic precursor population. *Blood*, **77**: 2122–8.

Smith, D.M., Ness, M.J., Landmark, J.D., Haire, W.W. & Kessinger, A. (1990). Recurrent neurologic symptoms during peripheral stem cell apheresis in two patients with intracranial metastases. *J. Clin. Apheresis*, **5**: 70–3.

Socinski, M.A., Cannistra, S.A., Elias, A., Antman, K.H., Schnipper, L. & Griffin, J.D. (1988). Granuloctye macrophage colony stimulating factor expands the circulating haemopoietic progenitor cell compartment in man. *Lancet*, i: 1194–8.

Spooncer, E.S., Gallagher, J.T., Krizsa, F. & Dexter, T.M. (1983). Regulation of hemopoiesis in long term bone marrow culture. IV. Glycosaminoglycan synthesis and stimulation of haemopoiesis by b-D-xylosides. *J. Cell. Biol.*, **96**: 510–14.

Sutherland, H.J., Lansdorp, P.M., Henkelman, D.H., Eaves, A.C. & Eaves, C.J. (1990). Functional characterization of individual human hematopoietic stem cells cultured at limiting dilution on supportive marrow stromal layers. *Proc. Natl. Acad. Sci. USA*, **87**: 3584–8.

Takaue, Y., Watanabe, T., Kawano, Y. *et al.* (1989a). Isolation and storage of peripheral blood hematopoietic stem cells for autotransplantation into children with cancer. *Blood*, **74**: 1245–51.

Takaue, Y., Watanabe, T., Kawano, Y. *et al.* (1989b). Sustained cytopenia after leukapheresis for collection of peripheral blood stem cells in small children. *Vox Sang.*, **57**: 168–71.

Tarella, C., Ferrero, D., Bregni, M. *et al.* (1991). Peripheral blood expansion of early progenitor cells after high-dose cyclophosphamide and rhGM-CSF. *Eur. J. Cancer*, **27**: 22–7.

To, L.B. (1990). Assaying the CFU-GM in blood: correlation between cell dose and haemopoietic reconstitution. *Bone Marrow Transplant.*, **5** (suppl. 1): 16–18.

To, L.B., Dyson, P.G. & Juttner, C.A. (1986). Cell-dose effect in circulating stem cell autografting. *Lancet*, ii: 404–405 (letter).

To, L.B., Haylock, D.N., Dyson, P.G., Thorp, D., Roberts, M.M. & Juttner, C.A. (1990b). An unusual pattern of hemopoietic reconstitution in patients with acute myeloid leukemia transplanted with autologous recovery phase peripheral blood. *Bone Marrow Transplant.*, **6**: 109–14.

To, L.B., Haylock, D.N., Kimber, R.J. & Juttner, C.A. (1984). High levels of circulating haemopoietic stem cells in very early remission from acute non-lymphoblastic leukaemia and their collection and cryopreservation. *Br. J. Haematol.*, **58**, 399–410.

To, L.B., Haylock, D.N., Thorp, D. *et al.* (1989). The optimization of collection of peripheral blood stem cells for autotransplantation in acute myeloid leukaemia. *Bone Marrow Transplant.*, **4**: 41–7.

To, L.B., Dyson, P.G., Ho, J.Q.K. *et al.* (1990a). APAAP- and flow cytometry-based CD34 measurements provide rapid indicators to determine the optimal time for recovery phase peripheral blood stem cell harvesting. *Blood*, **76** (suppl. 1): 569a (abstract).

To, L.B., Shepperd, K.M., Haylock, D.N. *et al.* (1990c). Single high doses of cyclophosphamide enable the collection of high numbers of hemopoietic stem cells from the peripheral blood. *Exp. Hematol.*, **18**: 442–7.

To, L.B., Haylock, D.N., Dyson, P.G. *et al.* (1992a). A comparison between 4 g/m² and 7 g/m² cyclophosphamide for peripheral blood stem cell mobilization *Int. J. Cell Cloning*, **10**: 33–5.

To, L.B., Roberts, M., Haylock, D.N. *et al.* (1992b). Comparison of haematological recovery times and supportive care requirements of autologous recovery phase peripheral blood stem cell transplants, autologous bone marrow transplants and allogeneic bone marrow transplants. *Bone Marrow Transplant.*, **9**: 277–84.

Verfaille, C., Blakolmer, K. & McGlave, P. (1990). Purified primitive human haemopoietic progenitors with long-term in vitro repopulating activity selectively adhere to irradiated bone marrow stroma. *J. Exp. Med.*, **172**: 509–20.

Vose, J.M., Kessinger, A., Bierman, P.J., Aharp, G., Garrison, L. & Armitage, J.O. (1992). The use of rhIL-3 for mobilization of peripheral blood stem cells in previously treated patients with lymphoid malignancies. *Int. J. Cell Cloning*, **10**: 62–5.

Williams, D.E. & Park, L.S. (1991). Hematopoietic effect of a granulocyte-macrophage colony-stimulating factor/interleukin-3 fusion protein. *Cancer*, **67**: 2705–7.

7

Minimal residual disease and blood stem cell transplants

J.G. SHARP AND A. KESSINGER

Introduction

The procedure for blood stem cell transplants is an evolving and rapidly growing alternative to autologous bone marrow transplants for the hematopoietic rescue of patients undergoing high dose therapy for cancer. There are two primary rationales for blood stem cell transplants as an alternative to autologous bone marrow transplants (Gale *et al.*, 1992a). One is the opportunity in at least some patient groups (mainly nonheavily pretreated patients) to achieve more rapid hematological recovery after high dose therapy with blood stem cell transplants than with autologous bone marrow transplants (Gianni *et al.*, 1990). The other reason, which has been a primary motivating factor in our program, is the notion, or at least the hypothesis, either that blood stem cell harvests may be less frequently contaminated with tumor cells than are autologous bone marrow harvests or that tumor cells shed from the primary tumor (or its metastases) into the circulation may be less able to reestablish tumor on reinfusion into patients than are tumor cells growing in marrow (Kessinger & Armitage, 1991). The initial evidence favoring this hypothesis is limited, but it has been difficult to establish primary tumors in culture, which suggests that only a few cells are clonogenic (Geara *et al.*, 1991; Masuda *et al.*, 1991). When tumor cells do grow, however, this indicates poor prognosis for survival (Masuda *et al.*, 1991; Sharp *et al.*, 1992a). The fact that patients early in the course of their disease generally either have no evidence of metastasis or have metastases only at limited sites is compatible with the idea that most tumor cells shed initially from the primary are unable to establish metastases (Mansi *et al.*, 1989). Experiments to test this hypothesis necessitate consideration of the question of whether tumor cells remaining in the patient after high dose therapy or tumor cells in the reinfused harvest are more likely contributors to relapse. It is also difficult to avoid the debate about the methodological considerations regarding the efficiency of detection of minimal residual disease in blood stem cell versus autologous bone marrow harvests.

Because of the relatively recent introduction of blood stem cell transplants as an alternative to autologous bone marrow transplants, or as an option for patients for whom an autologous bone marrow transplant is inappropriate or impossible, there is currently a limited amount of information about the importance of minimal residual disease to the outcome of blood stem cell transplants which can be used to evaluate these questions. This review attempts to present the concepts of minimal residual disease relevant to blood stem cell transplants, and to evaluate what is currently known about minimal residual disease and blood stem cell transplants and to identify questions which remain to be answered in future studies.

Minimal residual disease

What is minimal residual disease?

Although widely used and generally understood, the term minimal residual disease probably requires definition in the context of its use (Hagenbeek *et al.*, 1991). The definition we have adopted is that minimal residual disease exists when the tumor cells remaining in the patient after therapy or present in hematopoietic stem cell harvests, not detectable by either standard clinical or histopathologic techniques, respectively, may become a cause of relapse in the patient. According to this definition, a patient who achieves a complete clinical remission but subsequently relapses had residual disease even though he or she achieved a complete clinical remission. The fact that this disease was undetected defines it as minimal residual disease. Similarly, a bone marrow or blood stem cell harvest might appear to be normal when subjected to a standard histologic or cytologic analysis, but when subjected to more sensitive methods of tumor cell detection, such as molecular techniques, may be shown to contain tumor cells. We characterize this harvest as containing minimal residual disease.

The definition identifies two areas of concern. First, the adequacy of the cytoreductive regimen and its ability to eliminate minimal residual disease in the patient. This in turn leads to discussion of methods of detecting minimal residual disease, as the sensitivity of these methods improves, this, in turn, emphasizes the need for better cytoreductive regimens using either new agents, combinations of agents, dose intensification, or the combination of chemotherapy for cytoreduction with immunotherapy to attempt to eliminate minimal residual disease.

The second area of concern is the quality of the hematopoietic harvest and methods to assess 'quality'. If minimal residual disease is detected in the harvest should purging be employed? If so, how does one measure the efficacy of purging? Does purging harm the ability of the harvest to reconstitute the patient? In this context, some measure must be adopted to predict the ability of the harvest to reconstitute the patient, such as the number of mononuclear cells, granulocyte/macrophage colony-forming cells (GM-CFC), or CD34$^+$ cells (Siena *et al.*, 1991; Serke *et al.*, 1991). All of these are controversial topics. Increasing the volume of the harvest to ensure adequacy of reconstitution may also increase the risk of minimal residual disease in the harvest being transferred to the patient.

These areas of concern are relevant to both autologous bone marrow transplants and blood stem cell transplants. Much more information exists concerning minimal residual disease and autologous bone marrow transplants and it is useful to review this briefly before focusing on blood stem cell transplants.

Is minimal residual disease clinically relevant?

In a review of blood stem cell transplants, 'Past results and current prospects' by Abrams in 1983, minimal residual disease was not mentioned. At that time, the concerns were with obtaining successful reconstitution in diseases other than chronic myelogenous leukemia and the quality of reconstitution. In fact, inherent in early studies of the use of postchemotherapy rebound blood stem cell transplants in the acclerated phase of chronic myelogenous leukemia was the notion that not only was there an increased number of circulating progenitor cells (and by presumption, stem cells) but that the ratio of stem cell content to minimal residual disease might be much greater in such harvests than in bone marrow owing to reduction or elimination of circulating Philadelphia chromosome positive cells (Korbling *et al.*, 1981). The validity of these assumptions and their clinical relevance are still uncertain (Goldman, 1991), although some patients do better with this approach than would be expected for comparable patients treated by conventional therapy (Hughes *et al.*, 1991).

In 1983 also, in contrast to the situation in blood stem cell transplants, there was recognition of the potential need for purging of bone marrow for autologous bone marrow transplants and research into various techniques was in progress (Dicke, 1983). Despite the concerns about minimal residual disease in harvests leading to relapse, the value of purging of such harvests has only been established since about 1990. A number of studies have demonstrated that the presence of tumor cells at levels below histologic detection are associated with an increased risk of relapse in a number of cancers (Sharp & Crouse, 1992). It has been much more difficult, however, to demonstrate that purging these harvests is beneficial clinically. Recently, Gorin *et al.* (1991), reporting to the European registry, have shown a benefit of purging in acute myeloid leukemia. The same is true for acute lymphocytic leukemia (Miller *et al.*, 1991), and B cell lymphomas (Gribben *et al.*, 1991). If purging is beneficial for contaminated autologous bone marrow harvests then, by extrapolation, the same might be true for blood stem cell harvests, but there are technical considerations which cloud the issue. These are discussed later.

What are the methods of detection of minimal residual disease in blood stem cell harvests?

Currently the methods of detecting minimal residual disease in blood stem cell harvests are essentially the same as those employed to detect such disease in bone marrow harvests. The relative merits of those techniques have recently been extensively reviewed elsewhere (Sharp & Crouse, 1992). Briefly stated, for leukemias these involve detection of abnormal blasts on the basis of surface markers, oncogene over-expression or rearrangements and cytogenetics (Neale *et al.*, 1991; Roth & Terry, 1991; Yokota *et al.*, 1991). Lymphomas are best detected by clonal gene rearrangements and in low grade (t14:18) lymphomas by *bcl 2* rearrangements. Breast and other solid tumor cells (neuroblastoma, ovarian, etc.) are detected using morphologic and immunocytochemical methods. These methods can be applied directly or after a period of culture which attempts to amplify the tumor cells by maintaining or promoting their growth while permitting differentiated cells to complete their lifespan and die out (Sharp & Crouse, 1992).

The problems inherent in these approaches are the relative sensitivities of the techniques. Are these the same when applied to blood stem cell harvests versus autologous bone marrow harvests? One approach is to attempt to calibrate the systems by adding known and limiting numbers of tumor cells to the different types of harvest. When this is performed, the sensitivities seem similar (Sharp *et al.*, 1991). This approach, however, uses tumor cell lines with known characteristics and can be criticized as unrealistic. The morphologic/immunocytochemical techniques are open to the objection that a tumor cell growing in bone marrow may have a different degree of differentiation and therefore antigen expression (phenotype) than one shed directly into the circulation from the primary tumor and may therefore be more or less easily detectable (Gale *et al.*, 1992b). There is also a sampling problem in that it is not clear what is important: the relative number of tumor cells in the harvest, i.e. expressed per mononuclear cell or per stem cell, or the total number of tumor cells in the harvest? What about the 'quality' of the tumor cells, their clonogenicity or ability to reestablish tumor on transplantation? How do we measure these characteristics? Very different numbers of mononuclear cells are harvested and reinfused, containing very different frequencies of stem cells, from blood stem cell transplants and autologous bone marrow transplants, and it is currently impossible to make recommendations on theoretical grounds. We would prefer to adopt a pragmatic approach which requires investigators to demonstrate that their method of tumor cell detection is clinically relevant. This can be done by predicting the clinical outcome for a sample of patients. For example, we have studied retrospectively the outcome for a group of patients with breast cancer and other epithelial tumors whose blood stem cell transplant harvest was placed into culture and evaluated for the presence or absence of morphologically abnormal cells using methods described previously for bone marrow. The outcome appears poorer for those patients whose harvests contained abnormal cells in that only 1 of 5 is currently (1992) alive and disease free versus 10 of 23 of those whose harvest appeared normal (Sharp *et al.*, 1992b). Presumably, patients whose marrow and blood stem cell harvests are both contaminated with tumor cells are obvious candidates either for purging or for transplantation with separated, purified CD34$^+$ cells (Bensinger *et al.*, 1992).

Are blood stem cell harvests less frequently contaminated with relevant tumor cells than autologous bone marrow harvests?

This question can be divided into a number of subparts. Assume first of all that tumor cells in both types of harvest are equally able to reestablish tumor in the recipient. This leads to the following questions. Are blood stem cell harvests less frequently contaminated with such cells than are autologous bone marrow harvests or are such cells fewer in number in blood stem cell harvests? Alternatively, but not exclusively, are the tumor cells in blood stem cell harvests less able to reestablish tumor in the recipient than a similar number (see cautions above) in autologous bone marrow harvests?

Currently, not all of these questions can be answered by the data. In acute myelogenous leukemia, there is no difference in outcome from relapse between blood stem cell transplants and autologous bone marrow transplants. Morbidity, however, may be lower following blood stem cell transplants because of the reduction in the period of aplasia (Reiffers *et al.*, 1992).

In non-Hodgkin's lymphomas, Southern analysis of blood cells from patients is sometimes negative for clonal rearrangements even though these patients have clonal tumor in their marrow (Langlands *et al.*, 1990) and this has been confirmed employing the polymerase chain reaction (Langland *et al.*, 1992). Sensitive culture techniques which detect clinically relevant minimal residual disease in about 33% of autologous bone marrow harvests detect similar cells in only about 5% of blood stem cell transplant harvests (Sharp *et al.*, 1992b). These techniques have similar sensitivities when applied to the same number of cells sampled from the harvests as calibrated by T (CEM) and B (Raji) tumor cell lines added to normal harvests. Consequently, we conclude that non-Hodgkin's lymphoma tumor cells in blood stem cell harvests are present less frequently, or at lower levels (below the minimal level of sensitivity of the detection technique), or are less able to proliferate (required for detection by the culture technique) than are such cells in autologous bone marrow harvests. Also, in non-Hodgkin's lymphoma, patients with bone marrow involvement who undergo a blood stem cell transplant have a better outcome than patients without marrow involvement who undergo an autologous bone marrow transplant even if the autologous bone marrow harvest is apparently free from tumor cells (as defined by methods to detect minimal residual disease described earlier) (Sharp *et al.*, 1992b). Not surprisingly, autologous bone marrow transplant recipients with minimal residual disease in their marrow detected by sensitive techniques do worst of all (Sharp *et al.*, 1992a). This suggests that minimal residual disease in marrow is associated with a poor outcome just as is the case for minimal residual disease in blood stem cell harvests, as noted earlier for breast cancer and other solid tumors. Unfortunately, these observations have multiple potential explanations.

Clearly in acute myelogenous leukemia, blood stem cell harvests are as equally contaminated as autologous bone marrow harvests or, minimal residual disease in the patient is the primary cause of relapse and dominates any effects of minimal residual disease in the harvest. The simplest explanation for a better outcome of marrow positive non-Hodgkin's blood stem cell transplant patients compared with autologous bone marrow transplant recipients might be that the blood stem cell harvests are less contaminated with tumor cells. That would explain the different outcome compared with marrow minimal residual disease positive recipients but not, however, the better outcome compared with marrow minimal residual disease negative recipients. This implies that something else is happening. Perhaps blood stem cell harvests have an immunotherapeutic effect against minimal residual disease which is not present in marrow harvests? Immunologic effects of the transplant are important in the outcome of allografts for leukemia (Gale & Butturini, 1991). This raises the issue of what proportion of recurrences arise from tumor cells in the infused harvest versus tumor cells surviving at sites of bulk disease in the patients because nearly all relapses occur at sites of previous bulk disease. The group from the Dana–Farber Cancer Institute has recently reported that, following purged autologous bone marrow transplants for B cell lymphoma, some tumor cells inadvertently infused with the harvest may home to microenvironments at sites of original bulk disease and reestablish disease (Gribben *et al.*, 1991). We accept this possibility but have argued that recurrence from tumor cells surviving at sites of bulk disease is more probable (Sharp *et al.*, 1992b). Resolutions of this controversy may have to await the outcome of studies similar to those being performed by Brenner *et al.* (1992) in which the transplanted cells are marked by retroviral transfection. Unfortunately, because of current technical difficulties, the acquisition of patient data which prove to be informative may be slow. We have attempted an alternative approach, which is to compare the frequency of relapse in non-Hodgkin's lymphoma patients who receive an allotransplant with that in patients who receive an autotransplant. This is not a perfect approach because of the possible influence of graft-versus-lymphoma effects (Goldstone & Chopra, 1991). It assists us at least partly to partition the frequency of relapse between minimal residual disease in the harvest and minimal residual disease in the patients; the data are not yet mature but indicate that both are significant contributors. This leads to the conclusion that there is some evidence that blood stem cell transplants in non-Hodgkin's lymphoma are associated with a better outcome because the blood stem cell harvests are less likely to be contaminated with minimal residual disease than autologous bone marrow harvests, but this is far from a scientifically established fact.

In Hodgkin's disease, morphologically abnormal cells resembling Reed–Sternberg cells are detected by culture techniques more frequently in apheresis harvests than in bone marrow harvests. Statistically, these cells are highly associated with Hodgkin's disease and rarely observed in patients with other tumors. In addition to possessing all the relatively nonspecific (activation) markers associated with Reed–Sternberg cells, many of these cells are dually infected with multiple copies of Epstein–Barr virus and HHV-6 (human herpes) viruses. Potentially, the ability of these cells to grow in culture is associated with infection with these viruses. In the cultures, these cells appear early, by about 4 weeks, and are maintained and can dominate the cultures. Associated or derivative B cells in the cultures continue to amplify into cell lines. Clinically, the presence of these Reed–Sternberg like cells has no predictive value as to outcome (Sharp *et al.*, 1993). We postulate that these cells are a potential example of terminally differentiating malignant cells without the ability to transfer tumor to the host. They are associated with the long-term growth of B cells in culture and may be cytokine-producing cells which only amplify other cells in (micro)environments which they cannot reestablish on transplantation. They may be an artefact arising from virally-infected precursors. This serves, either way, to emphasize that not all cells which appear to represent minimal residual disease may be clinically significant.

Do cytokines employed to mobilize stem cells for collection also mobilize tumor cells?

There is evidence that cytokines can stimulate the growth of tumor cells. It is not surprising that growth factors for normal myeloid cells, e.g. GM-CSF, stimulate the replication of myeloid leukemic cells. Indeed, this may be exploited for therapeutic advantage (Valent *et al.*, 1990). What was, perhaps, unexpected is that some of these factors may influence the growth of epithelial tumor cells (Joraschkewitz *et al.*, 1990; Dippold *et al.*, 1991). This is a potentially greater problem when such factors are employed to increase the intensity of conventional doses of chemotherapy rather than in high dose therapy where the intent is to use tumor curative doses of chemotherapy. If the tumor is responsive to cytokines, the burden of minimal residual disease in the patient might be increased by pretherapy use of cytokines. A concern which is particularly relevant to the use of cytokines in blood stem cell transplants is that cytokines might mobilize tumor cells from sites of the primary disease and metastases (say in bone marrow) into the circulation in a manner analogous to that by which these factors mobilize stem cells into the blood. If this occurs, it will increase minimal residual disease in the harvest and potentially negate one of the advantages of blood stem cell transplants (see earlier). Presently, there are no reports of this occurring but it has been minimally studied. We have examined the IL-3 mobilized harvests of seven patients with Hodgkin's disease and two with non-Hodgkin's lymphoma and found no evidence of tumor cell mobilization or stimulation of tumor growth (Vose *et al.*, 1992). This requires additional investigation, however.

Summary

Minimal residual disease can exist both in hematopoietic harvests employed to reconstitute patients after high dose therapy and in the patient following therapy; both contribute to clinical outcome. In acute myeloid leukemia, minimal residual disease in the patient appears to be most important to outcome which is similar for blood stem cell transplants and autologous bone marrow transplants. Any advantage of blood stem cell transplants arises from shortening of the period of posttherapy aplasia.

In non-Hodgkin's lymphomas, minimal residual disease in the harvest is a very significant contributor as well as minimal residual disease in the patient, to outcome. Blood stem cell harvests in such patients appear to be contaminated less frequently with tumor than is bone marrow. There is evidence that this is clinically significant, because blood stem cell transplant recipients have a better survival than autologous bone marrow transplant recipients, although other factors may be involved.

In Hodgkin's disease, it is difficult to confirm that morphologically abnormal cells observed in blood stem cell or autologous bone marrow harvests are tumor cells, and the presence of such cells is not clinically important, although patients with histologically evident marrow disease have a poorer outcome than do patients without marrow involvement.

In breast cancer and other solid tumors, blood stem cell harvests may be somewhat less likely than autologous bone marrow harvests to contain minimal residual disease and such patients with marrow involvement undergoing blood stem cell transplants may do as well as patients undergoing autologous bone marrow transplants. Currently, there are insufficient data to critically evaluate the significance of minimal residual disease in blood stem cell transplants for solid tumors.

Acknowledgments

The investigators' research referred to in this report was supported in part by an Imogene Jacobs Memorial Grant from the American Cancer Society. We thank all members of the UNMC Transplant Team for making these studies possible and Roberta Anderson who typed the manuscript.

References

Abrams, R. (1983). Hematopoietic reconstitution using cells collected from the peripheral blood – Past results and current prospects. In *Recent Advances in Bone Marrow Transplantation*, ed. R.P. Gale, pp. 547–64. Alan R. Liss, New York.

Bensinger, W.I., Berenson, R.J., Andrews, R.G. *et al.* (1992). Engraftment after infusion of CD34 enriched marrow cells. *Int. J. Cell Cloning*, **10**: 176–8.

Brenner, M.K., Rill, D.R., Moen, R.C. *et al.* (1992). Applications of gene marking prior to autologous bone marrow transplantation. *J. Cell. Biochem.*, (abstract). **16A** (suppl. 1): 179.

Dicke, K.A. (1983). Purging of marrow cell suspensions. In *Recent Advances in Bone Marrow Transplantation*, ed. R.P. Gale, pp. 689–702. Alan R. Liss, New York.

Dippold, W.G., Klingel, R., Kerlin, M. *et al.* (1991). Stimulation of pancreas and gastric carcinoma cell growth by interleukin 3 and granulocyte-macrophage colony-stimulating factor. *Gastroenterology*, **100**: 1338–44.

Gale, R.P. & Butturini, A. (1991). How do bone marrow transplants cure leukemia? In *New Strategies in Bone Marrow Transplantation*, ed. R.E. Champlin & R.P. Gale, pp. 109–18. Wiley-Liss, New York.

Gale, R.P., Butturini, A. & Henon, P. (1992a). Is there a reason to use blood cell transplants? *Int. J. Cell Cloning*, **10**: 74–8.

Gale, R.P., Henon, P. & Juttner, C. (1992b). Blood stem cell transplants come of age. *Bone Marrow Transplant.*, **9**: 151–5.

Geara, F., Girinski, T.A., Chavaudra, N. *et al.* (1991). Estimation of clonogenic cell fraction in primary cultures derived from human squamous cell carcinomas. *Int. J. Radiat. Oncol. Biol. Phys.*, **21**: 661–5.

Gianni, A.M., Tarella, C., Siena, S. *et al.* (1990). Durable and complete hematopoietic reconstitution after autografting of rhGM-CSF exposed peripheral blood progenitor cells. *Bone Marrow Transplant.*, **6**: 143–5.

Goldman, J.M. (1991). Autografting for CML. Is there a role? *New Strategies in Bone Marrow Transplantation*, ed. R.E. Champlin & R.P. Gale, pp. 155–62. Wiley-Liss, New York.

Goldstone, A.H. & Chopra, R. (1991). Autografting in lymphoma: Prospects for the future. In *Autologous Bone Marrow Transplantation*, ed. K.A. Dicke, J.O. Armitage & M.J. Dicke-Evinger, 5th edn, pp. 551–62. University of Nebraska Medical Center, Omaha, NE.

Gorin, N.C., Labopin, M., Meloni, G. *et al.* (1991). Autologous bone marrow transplantation for acute myeloblastic leukemia in Europe: Further evidence of the role of marrow purging by Mafosfamide. *Leukemia*, **5**: 896–904.

Gribben, J.G., Freedman, A.S., Neuberg, D. *et al.* (1991). Immunologic purging of marrow assessed by PCR before autologous bone marrow transplantation for B-cell lymphoma. *N. Engl. J. Med.*, **325**: 1525–33.

Hagenbeek, A., Lu, Y-L, Arkesteijn, G.J.A., Ying, Y. & Martens, A.C.M. (1991). Minimal residual disease in acute leukemia: preclinical studies. *New Strategies in Bone Marrow Transplantation*, ed. R.E. Champlin & R.P. Gale, pp. 193–9. Wiley-Liss, New York.

Hughes, T.P., Brito-Babapulle, F., Tollit, D.J. *et al.* (1991). Induction of Philadelphia-negative hemopoiesis and prolongation of chronic phase in patients with chronic myeloid leukemia treated with high dose chemotherapy and transfusion of peripheral blood stem cells. *Autologous Bone Marrow Transplantation*, ed. K.A. Dicke, J.O. Armitage & M.J. Dicke-Evinger, 5th edn, pp. 219–28. University of Nebraska Medical Center, Omaha, NE.

Joraschkewitz, M., Depenbrock, H., Freund, M. *et al.* (1990). Effects of cytokines on in vitro colony formation of primary human tumor specimens. *Eur. J. Cancer*, **26**: 1070–4.

Kessinger, A. & Armitage, J.O. (1991). The evolving role of autologous peripheral stem cell transplantation following high-dose therapy for malignancies. *Blood*, **77**: 211–13.

Korbling, M., Burke, P., Braine, H., Elfenbein, G., Santos, G. & Kaizer, H. (1981). Successful engraftment of blood derived normal hemopoietic stem cells in chronic myelogenous leukemia. *Exp. Hematol.*, **9**: 684–90.

Langlands, K., Anderson, J.S., Parker, A.C. & Anthony, R.S. (1992). Polymerase chain reaction analysis of tumour contamination in peripheral blood stem cell harvests. *Int. J. Cell Cloning*, **10**: 95–7.

Langlands, K., Craig, J.I.O. & Parker, A.C. (1990). Molecular determination of minimal residual disease in peripheral blood stem cell harvests. *Bone Marrow Transplant.*, **5**: 64–5.

Mansi, J.L., Berger, U., McDonnell, T. *et al.* (1989). The fate of bone marrow micrometastases in patients with primary breast cancer. *J. Clin. Oncol.*, **7**: 445–9.

Masuda, N., Fukuoka, M., Matsui, K. *et al.* (1991). Establishment of tumor cell lines as an independent prognostic factor for survival time in patients with small-cell lung cancer. *J. Natl. Cancer Inst.*, **83**: 1743–8.

Miller, C.B., Zehnbauer, B.A., Piantadosi, S., Rowley, S.D. & Jones, R.J. (1991) Correlation of occult clonogenic leukemia drug sensitivity with relapse after autologous bone marrow transplantation. *Blood*, **78**: 1125–31.

Neale, G.A., Menarguez, J., Kitchingman, G.R. *et al.* (1991). Detection of minimal residual disease in T cell acute lympholastic leukemia using polymerase chain reaction predicts impending relapse. *Blood*, **78**: 739–47.

Reiffers, J., Korbling, M., Labopin, M., Henon, Ph. & Gorin, N.C. (1992). Autologous blood stem cell transplantation versus autologous bone marrow transplantation for acute myeloid leukemia in first complete remission. *Int. J. Cell Cloning*, **10**: 111–13.

Roth, M.S. & Terry, V.H. (1991). Application of the polymerase chain reaction for detection of minimal residual disease of hematologic malignances. *Henry Ford Hosp. Med. J.*, **39**: 112–16.

Serke, S., Sauberlich, S., Abe, Y. & Huhn, D. (1991). Analysis of CD34-positive hemopoietic progenitor cells from normal human adult peripheral blood: flow-cytometrical studies and in vitro colony (CFU-GM, BFU-E) assays. *Ann. Hematol.*, **62**: 45–53.

Sharp, J.G. & Crouse, D.A. (1992). Marrow contamination: detection and significance. In *High-Dose Cancer Therapy: Pharmacology, Hematopoietins and Stem Cells*, ed. J.O. Armitage & K.H. Antman, pp. 226–248. Williams & Wilkins, Baltimore, MD.

Sharp, J.G., Joshi, S.S., Armitage, J.O. *et al.* (1992a). Significance of detection of occult non-Hodgkin's lymphoma in histologically uninvolved bone marrow by a culture technique. *Blood*, **79**: 1074–80.

Sharp, J.G., Kessinger, A., Armitage, J.O. *et al.* (1993). Clinical significance of occult tumor cell contamination of hematopoietic harvests in non-Hodgkin's lymphoma and Hodgkin's disease. In *Autologous Bone Marrow Transplantation in Hodgkin's Disease, Non-Hodgkin's and Multiple Myeloma*, ed. A.L. Zander & B. Barlogie, pp. 123–132. Springer-Verlag, Berlin, Heidelberg.

Sharp, J.G., Kessinger, A., Vaughan, W.P. *et al.* (1992b). Detection and clinical significance of minimal tumor cell contamination of peripheral stem cell harvests. *Int. J. Cell Cloning*, **10**: 92–4.

Sharp, J.G., Vaughan, W.P., Kessinger, A. *et al.* (1991). Significance of detection
    of tumor cells in hematopoietic stem cell harvests of patients with breast
    cancer. In *Autologous Bone Marrow Transplantation*, ed. K.A. Dicke, J.O.
    Armitage & M.J. Dicke-Evinger, 5th edn, pp. 385–91. University of Nebraska
    Medical Center, Omaha, NE.
Siena, S., Bregni, M., Brando, B. *et al.* (1991). Flow cytometry for clinical
    estimation of circulating hematopoietic progenitors for autologous
    transplantation in cancer patients. *Blood*, 77: 400–9.
Valent, P., Geissler, K., Sillaber, C., Lechner, K. & Bettelheim, P. (1990). Why
    clinicians should be interested in interleukin-3. *Blut*, 61: 338–45.
Vose, J.M., Kessinger, A., Bierman, P.J., Sharp, G., Garrison, L. & Armitage,
    J.O. (1992). The use of rhIL-3 for mobilization of peripheral blood stem cells
    in previously treated patients with lymphoid malignancies. *Int. J. Cell Cloning*,
    10: 62–4.
Yokota, S., Hansen-Hagge, T.E., Ludwig, W.D. *et al.* (1991). Use of polymerase
    chain reactions to monitor minimal residual disease in acute lymphoblastic
    leukemia patients. *Blood*, 77: 331–9.

8

Blood versus bone marrow transplants

M. KORBLING, C. JUTTNER, P. HENON AND A. KESSINGER

Introduction

There is increasing use of myeloablative therapy and autologous stem cell rescue in the management of a variety of malignant lymphohematopoietic disorders and solid tumors. Autologous blood stem cell transplants are now a treatment modality and since their introduction clinical research has mostly focused on the following aspects:

kinetics of hematopoietic reconstitution after autologous blood stem cell transplants

contamination of harvested blood mononuclear cells with clonogenic tumor cells

stem cell peripheralization to temporarily increase blood stem cell concentration for stem cell harvest

stability and sustainment of short- and long-term hematopoietic reconstitution after autologous blood stem cell transplants.

Practical aspects, such as easy access to circulating stem cells and feasibility of stem cell harvest in case of tumor cell infiltration or prior radiation at the pelvic site, are an obvious advantage of using the autologous blood stem cell transplant option but the more pathophysiologic aspects of autologous blood stem cell transplants, such as multilineage hematopoietic reconstitution, clonogenic tumor cell exchange between marrow and peripheral blood and the character of primitive circulating hematopoietic stem cells, are still subjects of research.

In this chapter we summarize some pathophysiologic and clinical characteristics of autologous blood stem cell transplants and compare them with autologous bone marrow transplants.

Blood-derived versus bone marrow-derived hematopoietic stem cells

Bone marrow and circulating stem cell pools are in dynamic equilibrium with 98% of all committed stem cells located in the marrow, but only 0.1% circulate at any given time (Fliedner & Steinbach, 1988). There is no doubt that circulating clonogenic precursor cells can completely reconstitute hematopoietic function after myeloablative therapy, but whether circulating stem cells can sustain hematopoiesis lifelong has not yet been answered under clinical conditions. Gene marking studies will eventually define the long-term fate of transplanted blood stem cells (Brenner *et al.*, 1992).

In animal experiments there is strong evidence that blood-derived stem cells repopulate hematopoiesis permanently. Sex mismatched allogeneic transplantation of blood stem cells in dogs leads to stable chimerism 10 years after transplant (Carbonell *et al.*, 1984; Testa *et al.* 1992). Animal studies also suggest that blood stem cell autografts produce more rapid lymphoid repopulation than bone marrow autografts (Appelbaum 1979). An increased rate of lymphoid reconstitution has been reported in humans (To *et al.*, 1987a) and may be important, given the probability that part of the anti-tumor effect of allogeneic bone marrow transplants results from an immunological graft-versus-tumor effect (Gale & Butturini, 1989). An increase in the number of natural killer cells or subsets of T cells early after autologous blood stem cell transplants may be associated with a graft-versus-tumor effect and the potential for manipulating these cells with interleukin-2 (IL-2) or other immunomodulatory agents such as cyclosporine or linomide may have a significant potential advantage.

The phenotype of blood stem cell populations and subpopulations is being characterized and compared with marrow stem cell populations. $CD34^+$ hematopoietic progenitor cells are present in the circulation at about one-tenth of marrow concentration, and the relative frequency of these cells and their subpopulations differs in peripheral blood compared with bone marrow (Bender *et al.*, 1991). In most recent immunophenotyping studies reported by Bender *et al.* (1992) and Brugger *et al.* (1992), a small portion of mobilized $CD34^+CD38^-DR^-$ cells observed in the peripheral blood suggests the existence of circulating blast colony-forming cells with long-term repopulating ability (Terstappen *et al.*, 1991).

Blood stem cell mobilization and collection

The major drawback of harvesting blood stem cells over that of bone marrow is the time it takes. Usually three to eight aphereses on a daily or alternate day basis are needed to achieve a blood stem cell autograft sufficient to guarantee safe engraftment. Other problems associated with multiple aphereses are the cryopreservation of large volumes of mononuclear cell suspensions with the need for appropriate storage space, and the retransfusion of considerable amounts of free hemoglobin and dimethyl-sulfoxide (DMSO) (5–10% of frozen cell suspension volume) (Kessinger *et al.*, 1990). Therefore, crucial for a more general acceptance of the autologous blood stem cell transplant approach is a drastic reduction in the number of aphereses needed.

Stem cell aphereses can be timed to coincide with a stem cell rebound phase for maximal collection of stem cells. Cyclophosphamide priming (7 g/m²) results in a 11–70-fold increase in peak blood colony-forming unit (CFU) concentration over the pretreatment level, although patients in whom low numbers of blood stem cells have been mobilized have also been observed. Most observations have been carried out in patients with relapsing or progressing disease or those extensively exposed to alkylating agents and/or radiotherapy (To *et al.*, 1990b). The disadvantages of chemotherapy priming, which appears to require high doses of chemother-apeutic agents, include the frequent occurrence of fever, infectious complications, and the occasional mortality during the pancytopenia which accompanies chemotherapy priming (To *et al.*, 1990b; Henon *et al.*, 1992b). In addition, the effect of chemotherapy priming on stem cell mobilization is less predictable and, therefore, aphereses and cryopreservation cannot be planned ahead. Single dose cyclophosphamide, the most efficient mobilizing chemotherapeutic agent, is not generally considered to have a major anti-tumor effect, although chemotherapy priming has an additional *in vivo* purging effect.

Data on granulocyte-macrophage colony-stimulating factor (GM-CSF) mobilization of hematopoietic stem cells were first reported by Socinski *et al.* (1988). GM-CSF given alone significantly increased the number of circulating stem cells (an 18-fold increase). When GM-CSF was given during the leukocyte recovery phase following transient myelosuppression, the number of circulating CFU-GM rose to 62.5 times the pretreatment counts and five times the peak CFU-GM concentration seen after chemotherapy alone. Similar data were reported by Gianni *et al.* (1989), with an 80–550-fold increase in peak CFU-GM blood concentration after cyclophosphamide (7 g/m²) and GM-CSF in patients with solid tumors. Peak CFU-GM blood concentration increased to a median of 58-fold over pretreatment values with G-CSF application (Sheridan *et al.*, 1992). Most recently, sequential administration of IL-3 and GM-CSF was proposed by Brugger *et al.* (1992) for stem cell mobilization. Compared with GM-CSF alone, the combined administration of IL-3 and GM-CSF significantly increased the number of multilineage CFU-GEMM and immature CD34$^+$ subpopulations such as CD33$^-$ HLA-DR$^-$ CD38$^-$.

Latest developments in stem cell peripheralization include the use of human c-*kit* ligand or stem cell factor. When given to baboons, significant increases in circulating CFU and CD34$^+$ cells were seen (Andrews *et al.*, 1991). There is supposedly an expansion of both the marrow and the circulating stem cell pools.

The field is at an early stage in assessing mobilization by cytokines alone. Combined cytokine treatment (Moore, 1991) or the use of GM-CSF/IL-3 fusion protein PIXY 321 (Williams & Park, 1991) may be the most efficient way to transiently peripheralize stem cells for harvesting. Under optimal conditions, which include patients with no major marrow tumor cell infiltration and minor prior myelosuppressive treatment and with chemotherapy priming and/or cytokine treatment, one single apheresis is sufficient to recruit a functional blood stem cell autograft (M. Korbling, personal observation; Pettengell *et al.*, 1992).

The physical and technical aspects of blood stem cell apheresis are optimized and a number of studies have shown collection efficiencies in the 60–70% range. Consideration of nonmachine-related determinants suggests that it will be very difficult to further increase the collection efficiency (Keilholz *et al.*, 1991; Haylock *et al.*, 1992). Successful blood stem cell rescue has been performed using cells collected with a variety of cell separators, although those that are continuous flow in operation are less likely to cause circulatory instability during the collection process and those that are computer controlled are more likely to yield satisfactory results with a wide range of operators, including those who perform blood stem cell collections only occasionally.

Bone marrow collection and cryopreservation is clearly simpler. A single procedure is usually adequate with 800–1500 ml of bone marrow being aspirated from the pelvis and/or sternum by multiple punctures. The aspirated bone marrow is often screened for bone fragments and may be concentrated using density gradients, possibly using automated techniques. Problems of excessive volume and DMSO toxicity are much less significant.

Residual tumor cells in blood versus bone marrow

Since the advent of blood stem cell transplants it has been hypothesized that blood stem cells might be less contaminated by residual clonogenic tumor cells than are bone marrow cells, and therefore the risk of relapse after blood stem cell transplants might be less. There is still no definite evidence to prove the hypothesis, which mainly originated from the observation that in malignant lymphohematopoietic disorders the appearance of relapse is first seen in the marrow and somewhat later in the peripheral blood. Analysis of residual tumor cells is currently performed by studying gene rearrangements, by cytogenetics, PCR (polymerase chain reaction) and FISH (fluorescence *in situ* hybridization), and by long-term tumor cell cultures (Sharp *et al.*, 1991). Most data reported so far are based on steady state conditions, which may not be applicable during blood stem cell harvesting because of the multiple apheresis procedures, the use of cytokines or the use of chemotherapy-induced stem cell rebound. Tumor cell contamination in the blood stem cell population might be increased by the above mentioned perturbations of the hematopoietic system, but might also be decreased during early recovery from bone marrow aplasia, as reported by Carella *et al.* (1992) for chronic myelogenous leukemia and To *et al.* (1987b) for acute myeloid leukemia.

Number of stem cells required for safe engraftment

Quantitative assessment of the blood stem cell autograft is difficult. Some authors recommend target mononuclear cell numbers of 6×10^8/kg body weight for unmobilized cells (Kessinger *et al.*, 1991), whereas others emphasize the quantitative CFU-GM assay as a more useful stem cell indicator for predicting repopulating ability with mobilized cells (To *et al.*, 1990a). Unfortunately, the short-term CFU culture system is highly variable because of different growth conditions between various laboratories.

More recently, CD34$^+$ cells have been introduced as an indicator for stem cells and have been correlated with CFU-GM (Siena *et al.*, 1989). CD34$^+$ determination by flow cytometry is still difficult to perform because of low blood concentration in a high background (Bender & van Epps, 1991); however, the rapid assessment of total CD34$^+$ cell numbers may lead to a more usable 'real time' measure of stem cell levels in blood stem cell collections (Siena *et al.*, 1991). Highly mobilized stem cell products are expected to have CD34$^+$ cells and CD34$^+$ subpopulations large enough to make a precise phenotypic assessment. Gianni *et al.* (1989) have suggested that 8×10^6 CD34$^+$ blood cells /kg body weight will produce rapid and sustained engraftment. Berenson *et al.* (1991), on the other hand, using the biotin-avidin immunoadherence technique for purifying bone marrow CD34$^+$ cells, have proposed a marrow CD34$^+$ cell dose of 1×10^6/kg body weight.

Clinical studies of autologous blood stem cell transplants versus autologous bone marrow transplants

Prospective randomized trials to evaluate the kinetics of hematopoietic reconstitution and disease-free survival after autologous blood stem cell transplants compared with autologous bone marrow transplants have not been reported. Reiffers *et al.* (1992) retrospectively analyzed the data of the European Bone Marrow Transplant Registry Group (EBMTG) for acute myeloid leukemia patients transplanted in first complete remission. Patients receiving autologous blood stem cell transplants were compared with autologous bone marrow transplant patients or patients who had purged autologous marrow grafts and were matched for age, FAB subclassification and interval between complete remission and transplant. The actuarial risk of relapse was not significantly different for autologous blood stem cell transplant, autologous bone marrow transplant and purged autologous marrow graft patient cohorts, whereas the median number of days to reach 0.5×10^9 PMN (polymorphonuclear leucocyte) per liter of peripheral blood after transplant was significantly less in the autologous blood stem cell transplant patient group. Platelet reconstitution was not found to be different.

Registry data are based on rather heterogeneous transplant regimens, and therefore limited in their interpretation. In a single institution study (Korbling *et al.*, 1991), the kinetics of hematopoietic reconstitution and disease-free survival after autologous blood stem cell transplants in 20 patients were compared with autologous bone marrow transplants using Mafosfamide-purged marrow in 23 patients. All transplants were performed in first complete remission of acute myeloid leukemia under mostly standardized conditions. WBC (white blood cell) and PMN reconstitution after myeloablative therapy and stem cell transplants occurred significantly earlier, but with only borderline significance in favor of autologous blood stem cell transplants for platelet reconstitution. The patients' hospital stay was significantly shorter following autologous blood stem cell transplants compared with purged pautologous bone marrow transplants. The probability of disease-free survival 2 years after transplantation was higher in the purged pautologous bone marrow transplant group (51%) compared with the autologous blood stem cell transplant group (35%). The difference was not statistically significant because of the small sample size and limited statistical power. The autologous blood stem cell transplant group nevertheless lacked a stable disease-free survival plateau with relapses occurring more than 1 year posttransplant, which is unusual in autologous bone marrow transplants.

A preliminary evaluation of an ongoing prospective randomized trial (EBMTG study) (Reiffers *et al.*, 1992) in acute myelogenous leukemia patients assigned to receive an autologous blood stem cell transplant compared with an unpurged autologous bone marrow transplant did not reveal a significant difference in the probability of relapse.

A collaborative phase II autologous blood stem cell transplant study reported by Szer *et al.* (1992) was associated with even more rapid hematopoietic reconstitution and an actuarial disease-free survival of 38% at 26 months, equivalent to the two studies mentioned above. The period of hospitalization was even shorter for the Heidelberg group reported by Korbling *et al.* (1991). Hematopoietic reconstitution was not completely predictable, however, and there was a wide range in time to recovery, particularly for platelet reconstitution (Reiffers *et al.*, 1992). This may reflect differences in the quality of mobilized blood stem cells in acute myeloid leukemia compared with nonmyeloid malignancies and may result from acute myeloid leukemia remission sometimes being a differentiation of the underlying malignant clone rather than true clonal deletion.

In chronic myelogenous leukemia, studies have generally used chronic phase blood stem cells which are Ph-positive. It is interesting that a proportion of patients transplanted with chronic phase chronic myelogenous leukemia blood stem cells do develop partial or complete Ph negativity posttransplant, suggesting that the chronic phase cells contain a proportion of Ph-negative 'normal' long-term reconstituting cells (Butturini *et al.*, 1990). New stem cell purification techniques such as biotin-avidin immunoadherence (Berenson *et al.*, 1991), immunomagnetobead separation using directly conjugated $CD34^+$ beads (Egeland *et al.*, 1992), cell sorting or a combination of the above allow selection of putative 'normal' stem cells that are reported $CD34^+$ lineage$^-$ HLA-DR$^-$ (Verfaillie, 1992). In the chronic phase of chronic myelogenous leukemia they may permit exploration of autografting with these Ph$^-$ cells.

The published results in lymphoma mostly use steady phase or chemotherapy-primed blood stem cells collected from patients with bone marrow involvement with lymphoma or with irradiated bone marrow sites (Kessinger *et al.*, 1989; Korbling *et al.*, 1990). The preliminary results suggest no disadvantage for blood stem cells from marrow involved cases, with disease-free survival better than autologous bone marrow transplants using bone marrow cells from patients without overt marrow involvement in non-Hodgkin's lymphoma. In Hodgkin's disease the results are equivalent. In breast cancer and solid tumors, blood stem cells have mostly been used as an adjunct to autologous bone marrow transplants with the major aim of reducing the period of cytopenia and hospitalization, although blood stem cells have been used alone in breast cancer with bone marrow involvement (Kessinger *et al.*, 1986). The patient numbers and period of follow-up are still inadequate for other than preliminary conclusions at this stage. In multiple myeloma, blood stem cell autografting has been used as a technique to minimize tumor cell contamination using blood stem cells alone (Henon *et al.*, 1988; Fermand *et al.*, 1989; Ventura *et al.*, 1990) and in combination with bone marrow to expedite the rate of hematopoietic reconstitution seen with bone marrow alone.

Indications for autologous blood stem cell transplants versus autologous bone marrow transplants

It is still too early to define a panel of clinical indications for an autologous blood stem cell transplant being the preferred option over an autologous bone marrow transplant. An autologous blood stem cell transplant, as mentioned above is considered in cases where the pelvis has received prior irradiation which makes it unfeasible to harvest sufficient amounts of marrow stem cells (Kessinger *et al.*, 1989; Korbling *et al.*, 1990), or in cases with marrow tumor cell infiltration. The latter situation, although often proclaimed as an indication for an autologous blood stem cell transplant, might also coincide with tumor cell contamination of circulating mononuclear cells. Besides these well-defined indications, there is meanwhile some consensus that autologous blood stem cell transplants might be superior to autologous bone marrow transplants in patients where marrow tumor cell infiltration is high, such as in advanced breast cancer or in multiple myeloma, whereas the bone marrow option using a purged marrow autograft is preferred in patients with minimal residual disease. Both positive stem cell purification and negative tumor cell purging will, nevertheless, eventually be applied to blood stem cell as well as to bone marrow transplant approaches.

Some preliminary studies of cost analysis have been reported. Significant reductions in hospitalization are frequently but not universally seen (Korbling *et al.*, 1991; Henon *et al.*, 1992b; Sheridan *et al.*, 1992). The cost analysis must include the costs associated with mobilization and collection but, even allowing for this, there appears to be cost advantage for an autologous blood stem cell transplant, either alone or in combination with bone marrow. Briefer hospitalization has the potential to allow more patients to be transplanted in the limited number of beds available to most transplant units.

Conclusions and future aspects

The potential of autologous blood stem cell transplants is still being explored and is not limited to stem cell rescue in malignant lymphohematopoietic disorders. The shortening of total aplasia immediately after myeloablative therapy and stem cell transplantation with committed stem cells is the most striking advantage of autologous blood stem cell transplants over autologous bone marrow transplants. Further reduction in the period of aplasia may allow repeated myeloablative treatment cycles in solid tumors, an attractive treatment option for the further study of dose intensification.

More effective cytokine-induced mobilization of stem cells using IL-3 and GM-CSF/G-CSF or a combination of SCF, IL-1, IL-3 and GM-CSF/G-CSF might temporarily expand the circulating stem cell pool to an extent exceeding marrow stem cell concentration by 10–50-fold. This makes the more uniform blood stem cell population the ideal target for purification of $CD34^+$ cells or $CD34^+$ subpopulations to produce predictable short and long-term hematopoietic reconstitution.

References

Andrews, R.G., Knitter, G.H., Bartelmez, S.H. *et al.* (1991). Recombinant human stem cell factor, a c-kit ligand, stimulates hematopoiesis in primates. *Blood*, **78**: 1975–80.

Appelbaum, F.R. (1979). Hemopoietic reconstitution following autologous bone marrow and peripheral blood mononuclear cell infusions. *Exp. Hematol.*, **7** (suppl. 6): 7–11.

Bender, J.G., Williams, S.F., Myers, S., *et al.* (1992). Characterization of chemotherapy mobilized peripheral blood progenitor cells for use in autologous stem cell transplantation. *Bone Marrow Transplant.*, **10**: 281–5.

Bender, J.G., Unverzagt, K.L., Walker, D.E. *et al.* (1991). Identification and comparison of $CD34^+$ cells and their subpopulations from normal peripheral blood and bone marrow using multicolor flow cytometry. *Blood*, **77**: 2591–6.

Bender, J.G. & van Epps, D. (1991). Flow cytometric analysis of human bone marrow. In: *Bone Marrow Processing and Purging*, ed. A.P. Gee, pp. 137–54. CRC Press, Boca Raton, FL.

Berenson, R.J., Bensinger, W.I., Hill, R.S. *et al.* (1991). Engraftment after infusion of $CD34^+$ marrow cells in patients with breast cancer or neuroblastoma. *Blood*, **77**: 1717–22.

Brenner, M.K., Rill, D.R., Moen, R.C. *et al.* (1992). Applications of gene marking prior to autologous bone marrow transplantation. *J. Cell Biochem.*, **16A**: 179 (abstract DO29).

Brugger, W., Bross, K., Frisch, J. *et al.* (1992). Mobilization of peripheral blood progenitor cells by sequential administration of interleukin-3 and granulocyte-macrophage colony-stimulating factor following polychemotherapy with etoposide, ifosfamide and cisplatin. *Blood*, **79**: 1193–1200.

Butturini, A., Keating, A., Goldman, J. & Gale, R.P. (1990). Autotransplants in chronic myelogenous leukaemia: strategies and results. *Lancet*, **335**: 1255–8.

Carbonell, F., Calvo, W., Fliedner, T.M. *et al.* (1984). Cytogenetic studies in dogs after total body irradiation and allogeneic transfusion with cryopreserved blood mononuclear cells: observations in long-term chimeras. *Int. J. Cell Cloning*, **2**: 81–8.

Carella, A.M., Podesta, M., Carlier, P. *et al.* (1992). Conventional intensive therapy can lead to overshoot of Ph-negative blood cells in chronic myelogenous leukemia. *Int. J. Cell Cloning*, **10** (suppl. 1): 117–123.

Egeland, T., Quarsten, H., Gaudernack, G. (1992). Effect of recombinant stem cell growth factor on immunomagnetically isolated CD34$^+$ cells. *Int. J. Cell Cloning*, **10** (suppl. 1): 53–5.

Fermand, J.P., Levy, Y., Gerotta, J. *et al.* (1989). Treatment of aggressive multiple myeloma by high-dose chemotherapy and total body irradiation followed by blood stem cell autologous graft. *Blood*, **73**: 20–3.

Fliedner, T.M. & Steinbach, K.H. (1988). Repopulating potential of hematopoietic precursor cells. *Blood Cells*, **14**: 393–410.

Gale, R.P. & Butturini, A. (1989). Autotransplants in leukemia. *Lancet*, **ii**: 315–18.

Gianni, A.M., Siena, S., Bregni, M. *et al.* (1989). Granulocyte-macrophage colony stimulating factor to harvest circulating haemopoietic stem cells for autotranplantation. *Lancet*, **2**: 580–5.

Haylock, D.N., Canty, A., Thorp, D. *et al.* (1992). A discrepancy between instantaneous and overall stem cell collection efficiency. *J. Clin. Apheresis*, **7**: 6–11.

Henon, Ph., Beck, G., Debecker, A. *et al.* (1988). Autograft using peripheral blood stem cells collected after high-dose melphalan in high risk multiple myeloma. *Br. J. Haematol.*, **70**: 254–5 (Correspondence).

Henon, Ph., Eisenmann, J.C., Beck-Wirth, G. Liana, H. (1992a). A two-phase intensive therapeutic approach in high risk myeloma: follow-up. *Int. J. Cell Cloning*, **10** (suppl. 1): 142–4.

Henon, Ph., Liang, H., Beck-Wirth, G. *et al.* (1992b). Comparison of hematopoietic and immune recovery after autologous bone marrow or blood stem cell transplants. *Bone Marrow Transplant.*, **9**: 285–91.

Keilholz, U., Klein, H., Korbling, M. *et al.* (1991). Peripheral blood mononuclear cell collection from patients undergoing adoptive immunotherapy or peripheral blood-derived stem cell transplantation and from healthy donors. *J. Clin. Apheresis*, **6**: 131–6.

Kessinger, A., Armitage, J.O., Landmark, J.D. & Weisenburger, D.D. (1986). Reconstitution of human hematopoietic function with autologous cryopreserved circulating stem cells. *Exp. Hematol.*, **14**: 192–6.

Kessinger, A., Armitage, J.O., Smith, D.M. *et al.* (1989). High-dose therapy and autologous peripheral blood stem cell transplantation for patients with lymphoma. *Blood*, **74**: 1260–5.

Kessinger, A., Schmit-Pokorny, K., Smith, D. & Armitage, J. (1990).

Cryopreservation and infusion of autologous peripheral blood stem cells. *Bone Marrow Transplant.*, **5** (suppl. 1): 25–7.

Kessinger, A., Bierman, P.J., Vose, J.M. & Armitage, J.O. (1991). High-dose cyclophosphamide, carmustine, and etoposide followed by autologous peripheral stem cell transplantation for patients with relapsed Hodgkin's disease. *Blood*, **77**: 2322–5.

Korbling, M., Holle, R., Haas, R. *et al.* (1990). Autologous blood stem cell transplantation in patients with advanced Hodgkin's disease and prior radiation to the pelvic site. *J. Clin. Oncol.*, **8**: 978–85.

Korbling, M., Fliedner, T.M., Holle, R. *et al.* (1991). Autologous blood stem cell (ABSCT) versus purged bone marrow transplantation (pABMT) in standard risk AML: influence of source and cell composition of the autograft on hemopoietic reconstitution and disease-free survival. *Bone Marrow Transplant.*, **7**: 343–9.

Moore, M.A.S. (1991). The future of cytokine combination therapy. *Cancer*, **67**: 2705–7.

Pettengell, R., Demuynck, H., Testa, N. & Dexter, T.M. (1992). The engraftment capacity of peripheral blood progenitor cells (PBPC) mobilised with chemotherapy ± G-CSF. *Int. J. Cell Cloning*, **10** (suppl. 1): 59–61.

Reiffers, J., Korbling, M., Labopin, M. *et al.* (1992). Autologous blood stem cell transplantation versus autologous bone marrow transplantation for acute myeloid leukemia in first complete remission. *Int. J. Cell Cloning*, **10** (suppl. 1): 111–13.

Sharp, J.G., Vaughn, W.P., Kessinger, A. *et al.* (1991). Significance of detection of tumor cells in hematopoietic stem cell harvests of patients with breast cancer. In: *Autologous Bone Marrow Transplantation*, ed. K.A. Dicke, J.O. Armitage, M.J. Dicke-Evinger, pp. 385–91. University of Nebraska Medical Center, Omaha, Nebraska.

Sheridan, W.P., Begley, C.G., Juttner, C.A. *et al.* (1992). Effect of peripheral blood progenitor cells mobilised by filgrastim (G-CSF) on platelet recovery after high dose chemotherapy. *Lancet*, **339**: 640–4.

Siena, S., Bregni, M., Brando, B. *et al.* (1989). Circulation of CD34[+] hematopoietic stem cells in the peripheral blood of high-dose cyclophosphamide treated patients: enhancement of intravenous recombinant human granulocyte-macrophage colony-stimulating factor. *Blood*, **74**: 1905–4.

Siena S., Bregni, M., Brando, B. *et al.* (1991). Flow cytometry for clinical estimation of circulating hematopoietic progenitors for autologous transplantation in cancer patients. *Blood*, **77**: 400–9.

Socinski, M.A., Cannistra, S.A., Elias, A. *et al.* (1988). Granulocyte-macrophage colony stimulating factor expands the circulating haematopoietic progenitor cell compartment in man. *Lancet*, **i**: 1194–8.

Szer, J., Juttner, C.A., To, L.B. *et al.* (1992). Post-remission therapy for acute myeloid leukemia with blood-derived stem cell transplantation. Results of a collaborative phase II trial. *Int. J. Cell Cloning*, **10** (suppl. 1): 114–16.

Terstappen, L.W.M.M., Huang, S., Safford, M. *et al.* (1991). Sequential generations of hematopoietic colonies derived from single nonlineage-committed CD34[+] CD38[−] progenitor cells. *Blood*, **77**: 1218–27.

Testa, N.G., Molineux, G., Hampson, I.N. *et al.* (1992). Comparative assessment and analysis of peripheral blood and bone marrow stem cells. *Int. J. Cell Cloning*, **10** (suppl. 1): 30–2.

To, L.B., Juttner, C.A., Stomski, F. *et al.* (1987a). Immune reconstitution

following peripheral blood stem cell autografting. *Bone Marrow Transplant.*,
2: 111–12 (correspondence).

To, L.B., Russel, J., Moore, S., & Juttner, C.A. (1987b). Residual leukemia cannot
be detected in very early remission peripheral blood stem cell collections in
acute, non-lymphoblastic leukemia. *Leukemia Res.*, 11: 327–9.

To, L.B., Haylock, D.N., Dyson, P.G. *et al.* (1990a). An unusual pattern of
hemopoietic reconstitution in patients with myeloid leukemia transplanted
with autologous recovery phase peripheral blood. *Bone Marrow Transplant.*,
6: 109–14.

To, L.B., Shepperd, K.M., Haylock, D.N. *et al.* (1990b). Single high doses of
cyclophosphamide enable the collection of high numbers of hemopoietic stem
cells from the peripheral blood. *Exp. Hematol.*, 18: 442–7.

Ventura, G.J., Barlogie, B., Hester, J.P. *et al.* (1990). High dose of
cyclophosphamide, BCNU and VP-16 with autologous blood stem cell
support for refractory multiple myeloma. *Bone Marrow Transplant.*, 5: 265–8.

Verfaillie, C.M., Miller, W.J., Boylan, K. & McGlave, P.B. (1992). Selection of
benign primitive hematopoietic progenitors in chronic myelogenous leukemia
on the basis of HLA-DR antigen expression. *Blood*, 79: 1003.

Williams, D.E. & Park, L.S. (1991). Hematopoietic effects of a
granulocyte-macrophage colony-stimulating factor/interleukin-3 fusion
protein. *Cancer*, 67: 2705–7.

Part II
Clinical trials

9

Blood stem cell transplants in acute leukemia

C.A. JUTTNER

Introduction

Initial interest in autologous blood stem cell transplants in acute myeloid leukemia was based on the postulate that there might be less malignant contamination of blood stem cells than bone marrow stem cells (To *et al.*, 1984). The additional advantage of rapid hematopoietic reconstitution was immediately recognized with the initial application of clinical autologous blood stem cell transplants using mobilized cells (Juttner *et al.*, 1985; Korbling *et al.*, 1986; Reiffers *et al.*, 1986). This then led to the further postulate that rapid hematopoietic reconstitution might allow safer high dose therapy and autologous rescue, with shorter periods of hospitalization, lower cost, and the potential to offer intensive treatment to older patients than was currently the case with both allogeneic and autologous bone marrow transplants (To & Juttner, 1987). Other potential advantages were proposed, including collection in patients with bone marrow involvement by malignancy (probably not of relevance in acute leukaemia) (Kessinger *et al.*, 1986), collection without general anesthesia, collection after previous radiation therapy to the pelvic or sternal bones (of potential value in secondary acute myeloid leukemia following radiation therapy for Hodgkin's disease or non-Hodgkin's lymphoma, but not yet reported) and, finally, collection in the presence of bone marrow fibrosis (probably not relevant in acute myeloid leukemia as fibrosis at diagnosis is usually associated with reversal of the fibrosis after the achievement of remission with chemotherapy).

Most reported studies involve acute myeloid leukemia although there is an important case report of an allogeneic blood stem cell transplant in acute lymphoblastic leukemia using steady phase cells collected by ten aphereses from a sibling donor who was unwilling to have bone marrow harvested. Nine of the ten aphereses were depleted of T lymphocytes in an attempt to prevent graft-versus-host disease. There was initial evidence of engraftment, confirmed to be of donor origin by cytogenetic studies, but the recipient unfortunately died of sepsis and renal failure on day 32 after transplantation before either long-term hematopoietic reconstitution or long-term tumor response could be assessed (Kessinger *et al.*, 1989).

This chapter concentrates on acute myeloid leukemia and in particular on three published studies with adequate numbers of cases and sufficient follow-up to allow some conclusions to be drawn.

The design and characteristics of the three studies warrant further description. Korbling *et al.* (1991) reported 43 patients with acute myeloid leukemia transplanted in first complete remission. Seventy-five per cent of the patients were referrals from major German hematology/oncology centers, 25% were newly diagnosed at the Heidelberg Transplant Center and were followed from the beginning of their disease. Patients received blood stem cell or bone marrow autografts according to when they were included in the study, the blood stem cell autografts being performed on later patients. Reiffers *et al.* (1992) reported a study on behalf of the European Bone Marrow Transplant Registry (EBMT) group working party on autologous bone marrow transplants. Twenty-eight patients received blood stem cells and 683 patients received purged or unpurged autologous bone marrow transplants (study 1). A further analysis compared the results of blood stem cell autotransplants with those of twice as many patients from the EBMT Registry undergoing autologous bone marrow transplants or purged autologous bone marrow transplants who were matched for age, FAB (French, American, British) subclassification and the interval between complete remission and autotransplantation (study 2). In addition, Reiffers *et al.* briefly reported the preliminary results of a prospective Bordeaux, Grenoble, Marseilles and Toulouse study, where 32 patients were assigned to receive autologous transplants. Seventeen received unpurged autologous bone marrow transplants and ten received blood stem cells. Szer *et al.* (1992) reported the results of a phase II study of first remission blood stem cell autografting in 36 patients from six collaborating centres in Australia. The study design aimed at very early remission collection of blood stem cells with the potential for second rounds of collection after the first consolidation treatment. High dose therapy and autograft were also planned to be early (by 3 months postremission) to avoid time censoring by excluding patients who relapsed early before high dose therapy and transplants. Consecutive patients up to the age of 70 years were included in each participating center. There was an emphasis on standardization of the criteria for blood stem cell collection, of the granulocyte-macrophage colony-forming unit (CFU-GM) assays, and of the cryopreservation technique.

In all cases, blood stem cells were collected during hematological recovery in very early remission after induction chemotherapy or following consolidation chemotherapy. Bone marrow was collected later after the completion of consolidation. In Korbling's study, bone marrow was purged with maphosphamide at a concentration of 60–80 μg per 2×10^7 white blood cells, incubated at 37 °C for 30 min. Cells were then washed, resuspended with ABO compatible human plasma and cryopreserved at a final concentration of 10% DMSO (dimethylsulfoxide). In the EBMT group study, various forms of purging were used, most included maphosphamide in a range of doses. No attempt was made to purge any of the blood stem cell collections.

Table 9.1 shows patient demographics for the three studies. There were no significant differences in patient age, the male to female ratio, the time between the achievement of complete remission and transplant, the FAB subtype and the white cell count at diagnosis, although the Australian study did contain a high proportion of older patients.

Collection of bone marrow or blood stem cells

Table 9.2 shows the number of patients, the timing of collection, whether in early remission or after consolidation, the number of aphereses and the number of mononuclear cells and CFU-GM infused. Comparisons can be made between Korbling's and Szer's studies. In the Heidelberg study, more aphereses were performed, which probably explains the higher median number of mononuclear cells infused. Despite the higher number of mononuclear cells there was a significantly lower number of CFU-GM which may represent collection after more remission induction and consolidation chemotherapy, less emphasis on the timing of collection, or a less optimized CFU-GM assay than in Szer's study. The CFU-GM differences may explain the different pattern of hematopoietic reconstitution in the two studies. Reiffers' study does not provide mononuclear cell or CFU-GM numbers for either the blood stem cell or bone marrow autografts.

Hematopoietic reconstitution after high dose therapy

The high dose therapy used in Korbling's study consisted of cyclophosphamide (200 mg/kg body weight) and total body irradiation (14.4 Gy) in both the blood stem cell and autologous bone marrow transplant groups. In Reiffers' multi-institutional study, a variety of forms of high dose therapy were used. In Szer's study, all patients received bulsulphan (16 mg/kg) and cyclophosphamide (120 mg/kg).

Table 9.1. *Patient demographics: autologous transplants in acute myeloid leukemia*

	Korbling		Reiffers		Szer
	BSC	Purged ABMT	BSC	ABMT	BSC
No. of patients	20	23	28	683	36
Age years (range)	41 (5–48)	33 (17–50)	38 (18–50)	31 (1–62)	41 (10–68)
Sex (male/female)	12/8	14/9	NG	NG	19/17
CR→transplant (days)	105 (60–365)	122 (61–182)	159 (NG)	169 (NG)	90 (22–188)
FAB subtype					
M1	4	5	} 18	} 403	7
M2	5	2			11
M3	2	3			4
M4	7	9	} 10	} 280	8
M5	2	4			2
M6	—	—			2
M0					2
WCC at diagnosis $\times 10^9/l$	5.3(0.5–268)	17.6(0.7–277)	NG	NG	6.8(0.5–475)

ABMT, autologous bone marrow transplant; BSC, blood stem cell; CR, complete remission; FAB, French, American, British classification of leukemia; NG, not given; WCC, white cell count. Values are complete numbers of median (range).

Table 9.2. *Bone marrow and blood stem cell collection*

	Korbling		Reiffers		Szer
	BSC	Bone marrow	BSC	Bone marrow	BSC
No. of patients	20	23	28	683	36
Timing of collection					
Early remission	−	−	+	−	+
Post consolidation	+	+	+	+	+
No. of aphereses	10(6–14)	—	NG	—	5(3–10)
MNC ×10^8/kg infused	8(1.7–14.1)	0.4(0.06–1.3)	NG	NG	3.6(0.5–14)
CFU-GM ×10^4/kg infused	2.4(0.4–4.1)	0.14(0.006–1.0)	NG	NG	77(25–257)

MNC, mononuclear cells × 10^8/kg recipient body weight (median, range); CFU-GM, granulocyte-macrophage colony-forming units/kg recipient body weight (median, range); BSC, blood stem cell; NG, not given.

Table 9.3. *Initial hematopoietic reconstitution: blood stem cell versus bone marrow in acute myeloid leukemia first complete remission*

	Korbling		Reiffers		Szer
	BSC	Purged ABMT	BSC	ABMT	BSC
No. of patients	20	23	28	683	36
Days to 0.5 $\times 10^9$ PMN/l	14 (NG)	42 (NG)	15.5(9–60)	27(9–389)	11(9–16)
Days to 2.0 $\times 10^9$ PMN/l	–	–	–	–	14(10–24)
Days to 20 $\times 10^9$ platelets/l	30 (NG)	46 (NG)	–	–	–
Days to 50 $\times 10^9$ platelets/l	–	–	58.5(11–713)	50(10–700)	13(9–337)
Days to 150 $\times 10^9$ platelets/l	–	–	–	–	48(10–NR)
Early deaths	1	0	NG	NG	1
Days in hospital (median)	48 (NG)	73 (NG)	NG	NG	27(22–69)

BSC, blood stem cell; ABMT, autologous bone marrow transplant; PMN, polymorphonuclear leucocytes; NG, not given; NR, not reached.
Values are whole numbers or median (range).

Table 9.3 shows the initial hematopoietic reconstitution in the three studies. Neutrophil recovery to $0.5 \times 10^9/l$ was significantly faster after blood stem cell than after purged autologous bone marrow transplants in Korbling's study or after a mixture of purged or unpurged autologous bone marrow transplant in Reiffers' study. In Szer's study, similarly rapid neutrophil recovery was seen including the median time of 14 days (range 10–24 days), to achieve a normal neutrophil count of $2.0 \times 10^9/l$, which was as fast as the time to 0.5×10^9 neutrophils/l in both Korbling's and Reiffers' blood stem cell groups. Platelet recovery to $20 \times 10^9/l$ was faster in Korbling's blood stem cell group than in his purged autologous bone marrow transplant group. In Reiffers' study, platelet recovery to $50 \times 10^9/l$ was no faster in the blood stem cell group than the autologous bone marrow transplant group, whereas Szer reported recovery to a platelet count of $50 \times 10^9/l$ at a median of 13 days compared with a median of 30 days to recover to $20 \times 10^9/l$ for Korbling's patients receiving blood stem cells. These differences may result from the significantly higher number of blood stem cells (measured by the CFU-GM assay) infused in the collaborative Australian study.

There have been reports of a transient secondary fall in neutrophil and platelet counts after blood stem cell transplants in acute myeloid leukemia (To et al., 1990). The level of the secondary platelet nadir correlated with the CFU-GM dose infused but not with the mononuclear cell dose infused. There was no correlation between CFU-GM dose infused and the level of the secondary neutrophil nadir. Not all patients demonstrated the secondary fall, although more (12 of 14) had a fall in platelets than a fall in neutrophils (5 of 14). This group of patients were also examined in relation to the previously proposed safe minimum or threshold CFU-GM dose of 50×10^4 CFU-GM/kg body weight (To et al., 1986). All three patients who received $< 50 \times 10^4$ CFU-GM/kg had secondary neutrophil nadirs of $< 1.0 \times 10^9/l$ and secondary platelet nadirs of $< 25 \times 10^9/l$ whereas none of 11 receiving $> 50 \times 10^4$ CFU-GM/kg had neutrophil nadirs of $< 1.0 \times 10^9/l$ and only 4 of 11 had platelet nadirs of $< 25 \times 10^9/l$. It has been suggested that this resulted from a relative deficiency of intermediate and long-term repopulating cells in mobilized peripheral blood stem cell collections. Table 9.4 presents the data for longer term hematopoietic reconstitution from the Heidelberg and Australian first remission autograft studies. Korbling reported fewer patients with a platelet count of $< 20 \times 10^9/l$ at day 100 following blood stem cell autotransplants than after purged autologous bone marrow transplants. In Szer's study 1 of 32 patients had $< 20 \times 10^9/l$ platelets 3 months posttransplant, even though every patient achieved a

Table 9.4. *Later hematopoietic reconstitution: blood stem cells versus bone marrow*

	Korbling		Szer	
	BSC	Purged ABMT	BSC	
Platelets				
$<20 \times 10^9$/l at day 100, or 3 or 6 months	3/20 (day 100)	8/22 (day 100)	1/32 (3 months)	0/22 (6 months)
$<50 \times 10^9$/l at 3 or 6 months	NG	NG	5/32 (3 months)	2/22 (6 months)
$<150 \times 10^9$/l at 3 or 6 months	NG	NG	27/32 (3 months)	10/22 (6 months)
Polymorphonuclear leucocytes				
$<1.0 \times 10^9$/l at 3 or 6 months	NG	NG	0/32 (3 months)	0/22 (6 months)
$<2.0 \times 10^9$/l at day 100	NG	NG	9/32 (3 months)	7/22 (6 months)

BSC, blood stem cells; ABMT, autologous bone marrow transplant; NG, not given.

platelet count of $> 50 \times 10^9/l$ at median day 13 following transplantation. At 3 months, 5 of 32 assessable patients had $< 50 \times 10^9/l$ and 27 of 32 had $< 150 \times 10^9$ platelets/l. In the same study, 9 of 32 patients had not maintained the neutrophil count in the normal range ($> 2.0 \times 10^9/l$) at 3 months whereas all patients initially achieved this level by day 24. The results in Table 9.4 show that patients subsequently had gradual recovery towards normal counts in the absence of relapse. This larger study in first remission blood stem cell autografting confirms the transient nature of the secondary fall in peripheral blood counts previously reported in a smaller number of patients autografted in relapse or remission (To *et al.*, 1990).

Tumor response, relapse and disease-free survival

The results of these three first remission autografting studies are shown in Table 9.5. The greatest differences appear to lie between the blood stem cell and purged autologous bone marrow transplant group in Korbling's study. At the time of publication the median time to relapse had not been reached for the purged autologous bone marrow transplant group whereas the median time to relapse in the blood stem cell group was 8.1 months. The disease-free survival at 2 years was 35% for the blood stem cell group and 51% for the autologous bone marrow transplant group. None of these differences was statistically significant. In Reiffers' study the differences in actuarial risk of relapse and disease-free survival were not significantly different for the blood stem cell and autologous bone marrow transplant groups and the actuarial disease-free survival in the Australian collaborative study is remarkably similar to Korbling's and Reiffers' blood stem cell groups. Table 9.6 shows the results of Reiffers' study 2 with a comparison of blood stem cell autografts with twice the number of unpurged and purged autologous bone marrow transplant patients from within the EBMT database, matched for age, FAB subtype and the time from complete remission to transplant. No significant differences are seen. Reiffers also reported a prospective study where patients are randomized by geographic site of treatment. Thus, patients in Bordeaux received blood stem cell autografts and those in Grenoble, Marseilles or Toulouse received bone marrow autografts. Of 32 patients assigned for autologous transplants, 17 underwent autologous bone marrow transplants and 10 received blood stem cell transplants. At a median follow up of 22 months, five patients had leukemic relapse in each group and the disease-free survival was not significantly different. The tentative conclusion must be that blood stem cell autografting offers no advantages in leukemia-free survival over

Table 9.5. *Relapse of acute myeloid leukemia and disease-free survival*

	Korbling		Reiffers		Szer
	BSC	Purged ABMT	BSC	ABMT	BSC
No. of patients	20	23	28	683	36
Median time to relapse (months)	8.1	NR	NG	NG	13.5
Actuarial risk of relapse	NG	NG	57±10%	48±6%	NG
Disease-free survival	35±21% (2 years)	51±21% (2 years)	39±10% (time not stated)	42±5% (time not stated)	38±8% (26 months)

BSC, blood stem cell; ABMT, autologous bone marrow transplant; NR, not reached; NG, not given.
Actuarial risk of relapse and disease-free survival are shown as percentages ± standard error of mean.

Table 9.6. *Outcome of blood stem cells versus purged and unpurged autologous bone marrow transplants matched for age, FAB subtype and time from complete remission to transplant*

	BSC	ABMT	Purged ABMT
No. of patients	28	56	56
Age (range) years	40(20–70)	40(15–60)	35(15–60)
CR→transplant (days)	130(50–410)	130(60–440)	140(20–710)
Actuarial risk of relapse	57±10%	64±12%	50±10%
Actuarial DFS	39±10%	31±10%	39±6%

BSC, blood stem cell; ABMT, autologous bone marrow transplant; CR, complete remission; DFS, disease-free survival.

autologous bone marrow transplants, but the rate of hematopoietic reconstitution and duration of hospitalization may be better.

Blood stem cell autografts have not been extensively performed in more advanced acute myeloid leukemia. Reiffers, however, has reported 11 patients in second complete remission receiving recovery phase blood stem cells after either cyclophosphamide (120 mg/kg body weight) and total body irradiation or the combination of busulphan (16 mg/kg) and either cyclophosphamide or melphalan (Reiffers *et al.*, 1991). There was one early death, six patients relapsed and four were alive in continuing complete remission with a median follow-up of 2 years. In our own early experience, blood stem cell autografting was offered only to patients in acute myeloid leukemia relapse because of initial uncertainty about the hematopoietic reconstitutive capacity of these cells. Nine acute myeloid leukemia patients received high dose therapy and early remission blood stem cell autografts as initial therapy for first relapse after varying periods in unmaintained remission. One patient died of infection 65 days after autograft without evidence of relapse. The other eight patients all achieved a second complete remission but subsequently relapsed between 21 and 460 days after autograft (median 166 days). None of these patients received any further anti-leukemic therapy after autografting (C.A. Juttner *et al.*, unpublished data).

It is uncertain whether relapse after autografting is from failure of the high dose therapy to eradicate all the acute myeloid leukemia cells in the patient or to the infusion of clonogenic leukemic cells in the graft.

Malignant contamination

Initial case reports of blood stem cell transplants proposed reduced malignant contamination largely on a theoretical basis. The very early remission phase in acute leukemia may be associated with lower numbers of malignant cells because leukemic cells are known to proliferate less rapidly than normal cells (Arlin *et al.*, 1978; To *et al.*, 1984). Also, those cells might not circulate as readily as normal cells (McCarthy & Goldman, 1984). Data from studies of chronic myelogenous leukemia suggest that malignant cells in this disease are more likely to circulate than are normal cells, but similar studies are yet to be performed in acute myeloid leukemia, and increasing information on mechanisms of adhesion of normal and leukemic cells may yield further support for the postulate of reduced circulation of leukemic cells. Little firm data are available, although one study which examined acute myeloid leukemia patients with the (8;21) translocation demonstrated that leukemic colonies could be grown from cryopreserved leukemic cells, that the (8;21) translocation could be demonstrated in those colonies and that cryopreserved early remission blood stem cells from those patients revealed no (8;21) translocations in 293 metaphases examined (To *et al.*, 1987). Two patients subsequently received high dose therapy and autologous very early remission blood stem cell rescue at first relapse. Both patients achieved remission but neither of those remissions was durable, with relapse occurring 9 and 15 months following autotransplant. In a later report, Castagnola *et al.* (1989) reported that the karyotypic abnormality present at diagnosis in a patient with acute myeloid leukemia could be found in 30% of the metaphases from early remission peripheral blood cells collected by leukapheresis. Newer techniques in molecular genetics, including studies of H-*ras* mutations and fluorescence *in situ* hybridization, may yield more sensitive and specific results than those already published, but no information is yet available. There is also little certainty that relapse in autografting results from infused clonogenic cells, and the presence of a 20% relapse rate in acute myeloid leukemia in first complete remission after allogeneic bone marrow transplants and a 40–60% relapse rate after syngeneic bone marrow transplants suggests that residual leukemia in the patient after high dose therapy may be a greater problem than infused clonogenic leukemic cells.

Conclusion

The potential role of blood stem cell autografting as a new therapeutic option for acute myeloid leukemia was addressed in an annotation in the *British Journal of Haematology* in 1987 (To & Juttner, 1987). No prospective randomized studies are currently available. The three studies explored in detail in this review demonstrate possible advantages in that blood stem cell-transplants produce granulocyte reconstitution which is clearly faster than either purged or unpurged autologous bone marrow transplants. Also, platelet reconstitution may be faster depending on the dose of blood stem cells and when they are collected. There is less prolonged hospitalization with a probable associated reduction in cost and the potential for transplanting more patients per year with a set and limited number of beds. Szer's study suggests that blood stem cell transplants may allow a higher percentage of patients of advanced age to be treated with dose therapy and autologous rescue because 25% of the patients in his study were over the age of 60 years and 42% were over the age of 50 years. In addition, this study, in which patients appearing to be entering remission were enrolled on the basis of a rapidly rising platelet and/or neutrophil count, was associated with the ability to carry out planned high dose therapy and autotransplantation in the high proportion of 36 of 49 (73%) of all patients. Eight patients (16%) refused to proceed with the study, three patients (6%) had insufficient blood stem cells because of failure to collect the predetermined minimum level of 25×10^4 CFU-GM/kg, and two patients (4%) did not receive transplants because of persistent hepatosplenic candidiasis. There were no relapses before autologous blood stem cell transplants and thus no time disadvantage. This compares favorably with other studies where much lower numbers of remitting patients actually proceed to autotransplantation. In a study reported by Berman *et al.* (1991) only 4 of 24 (17%) eligible patients under the age of 50 years who achieved remission and were planned for autologous bone marrow transplants actually received autologous bone marrow transplants. In the current MRC-10 study all remitting patients receive four courses of intensive consolidation and then an allogeneic bone marrow transplant if an HLA-matched donor is available. The remainder are randomized to stop therapy or to receive an unpurged autologous bone marrow transplant. Burnett *et al.* (1991) presented preliminary data at the Fifth International Symposium on Autologous Bone Marrow Transplantation in Omaha in July 1990. In 299 patients who achieved remission, 52 had not reached the randomization point, 10 (3%) experienced early relapse and 12 (4%) died of sepsis during consolidation therapy. Sixty-three patients had an HLA-matched sibling and were allocated to allogeneic bone marrow transplants. A total of 162 patients were thus available for randomization. Seven of these (4%) elected to receive an autograft and 41 (25%) were not randomized for various reasons. There were 114 patients who were randomized to either early autograft ($n = 57$, 35%) or stop therapy ($n = 57$). This study is limited to patients under the age of 55 years, a policy which would have excluded 10 of the 36 patients (28%) in Szer's study who were all older than 55 years and were autografted without treatment-related mortality resulting.

The potential disadvantages of blood stem cell transplants include the possibility that relapse may be greater with blood stem cell transplants, particularly when compared with purged autologous bone marrow transplants although the differences in Korbling's study are not statistically significant. There is uncertainty about hematopoietic reconstitution and a lack of knowledge of definite criteria to predict both short-term and long-term hematopoietic reconstitution. Rapid platelet hematopoietic reconstitution in particular may require blood stem cell collection very early after remission induction or consolidation chemotherapy, at a time when *in vivo* purging by initial chemotherapy may be inadequate. Other disadvantages lie in the practicalities of multiple aphereses, the cryopreservation of large volumes of stem cells on multiple occasions (whereas autologous bone marrow requires only a single cryopreservation) and the subsequent potential toxicity of infusing large volumes of DMSO (Kessinger *et al.*, 1990). Hematopoietic growth factors, particularly recombinant human (rh)GM-CSF and rhG-CSF, demonstrated effective in increasing blood stem cell yields and hematopoietic reconstitution after high dose therapy and autotransplants (Gianni *et al.*, 1990; Sheridan *et al.*, 1992) cannot be applied in acute myeloid leukemia because of their potential to stimulate residual leukemic cells. The lack of sensitive and specific techniques to assess malignant contamination is a further problem for both autologous blood stem cell and bone marrow transplants.

Large prospectively randomized studies comparing chemotherapy, autologous bone marrow transplants and autologous blood stem transplants with careful assessment of mononuclear cell numbers, CFU-GM numbers and CD34[+] cell numbers are required. Follow-up should include assessment of early and late hematopoietic reconstitution, malignant contamination, morbidity and mortality during the transplant procedure, duration of hospitalization, the extent of support required, and the outcome in terms of relapse and disease-free survival. This must be seen in the context of current uncertainty on whether high dose therapy and autologous transplantation improves the outcome in acute myeloid leukemia, given the recent improvements in the results of relatively conventional dose chemotherapy in producing long-term disease-free survival and possible cure in up to 40% of remitters in some reports, although most large studies have long-term disease-free survival rates of 15–25%. Several reports suggest that the combination of relatively small numbers of blood stem cells with bone marrow may ensure satisfactory early and late hematopoietic reconstitution, and the Australian collaborative group is embarking on a study of combined bone marrow and blood stem cell autotransplants with both sources of stem cells collected later in the course of disease after intensive consolidation therapy. If this phase II study appears feasible, the Australian Leukemia Study Group may incorporate this approach as a second randomization in its next major study.

References

Arlin, Z.A., Fried, J. & Clarkson, B.D. (1978). Therapeutic role of cell kinetics in acute leukaemia. *Clin. Haematol.*, **7**: 339–62.
Berman, E., Heller, G. & Santorsa, J. (1991). Results of a randomized trial

comparing idarubicin and cytosine arabinoside with daunorubicin and cytosine arabinoside in adult patients with newly diagnosed acute myelogenous leukemia. *Blood*, 77: 1666–74.

Burnett, A.K., Goldstone, A.H., Hann, I.M. *et al.* (1991). Evaluation of autologous bone marrow transplantation in acute myeloid leukaemia: a progress report on the MRC 10th AML trial. In *Autologous Bone Marrow Transplantation. Proceedings of the Fifth International Symposium*, ed. K.A. Dicke, J.O. Armitage & M.J. Dicke-Evinger, pp. 3–7. University of Nebraska Medical Centre, Omaha.

Castagnola, C., Bonfichi, M., Colombo, A., Bernasconi, P. & Bernasconi, C. (1989). Acute nonlymphocytic leukemia: evidence of clonogenic cells in peripheral blood in early complete remission. *Acta Haematol.*, 82: 210–12.

Gianni, A.M., Tarella, C., Siena, S. *et al.* (1990). Durable and complete hematopoietic reconstitution after autografting of rhGM-CSF exposed peripheral blood progenitor cells. *Bone Marrow Transplant.*, 6: 143–5.

Juttner, C.A., To, L.B., Haylock, D.N., Branford, A. & Kimber, R.J. (1985). Circulating autologous stem cells collected in very early remission from acute non-lymphoblastic leukaemia produce prompt but incomplete haemopoietic reconstitution after high dose melphalan or supralethal chemoradiotherapy. *Br. J. Haematol.*, 61: 739–45.

Kessinger, A., Armitage, J.O., Landmark, J.D. & Weisenburger, D.D. (1986). Reconstitution of human hematopoietic function with autologous cryopreserved circulating stem cells. *Exp. Hematol.*, 14: 192–6.

Kessinger, A., Schmit-Pokorny, K., Smith, D. & Armitage, J. (1990). Cryopreservation and infusion of autologous peripheral blood stem cells. *Bone Marrow Transplant.*, 5 (suppl. 1): 25–7.

Kessinger, A., Smith, D.M., Strandjord, S.E. *et al.* (1989). Allogeneic transplantation of blood-derived, T cell-depleted hemopoietic stem cells after myeloablative treatment in a patient with acute lymphoblastic leukemia. *Bone Marrow Transplant.*, 4: 643–6.

Korbling, M., Dorken, B., Ho, A.D., Pezzuto, A., Hunstein, W. & Fliedner, T.M. (1986). Autologous transplantation of blood-derived hemopoietic stem cells after myeloablative therapy in a patient with Burkitt's lymphoma. *Blood*, 67: 529–32.

Korbling, M., Fliedner, T.M., Holle, R. *et al.* (1991). Autologous blood stem cell (ABSCT) versus purged bone marrow transplantation (pABMT) in standard risk AML: influence of source and cell composition of the autograft on hemopoietic reconstitution and disease-free survival. *Bone Marrow Transplant.*, 7: 343–9.

McCarthy, D.M. & Goldman, J.K. (1984). Transfusion of circulating stem cells. *CRC Crit. Rev. Clin. Lab. Sci.*, 20: 1–24.

Reiffers, J., Bernard, P., David, B. *et al.* (1986). Successful autologous transplantation with peripheral blood haemopoietic cells in a patient with acute leukaemia. *Exp. Hematol.*, 14: 312–15.

Reiffers, J., Korbling, M., Labopin, M., Henon, Ph., Gorin, N.C. on behalf of the EBMT Group Working Party for Autologous Bone Marrow Transplantation. (1992). Autologous blood stem cell transplantation versus autologous bone marrow transplantation for acute myeloid leukemia in first complete remission. *Int. J. Cell Cloning*, 10 (suppl. 1): 111–13.

Reiffers, J., Marit, G., Rice, A. *et al.* (1991). Peripheral blood stem cell transplantation in patients with acute myeloid leukemia. In *Autologous Bone*

116 *C.A. Juttner*

Marrow Transplantation. Proceedings of the Fifth International Symposium, ed. K.A. Dicke, J.O. Armitage and M.J. Dicke-Evinger, pp. 823–827. University of Nebraska Medical Centre, Omaha.

Sheridan, W.P., Begley, C.G., Juttner, C.A. *et al.* (1992). Effect of peripheral-blood progenitor cells mobilised by filgrastim (G-CSF) on platelet recovery after high-dose chemotherapy. *Lancet*, **339**: 640–4.

Szer, J., Juttner, C.A., To, L.B. *et al.* (1992). Post-remission therapy for acute myeloid leukaemia with blood-derived stem cell transplantation. Results of a collaborative Phase II trial. *Int. J. Cell Cloning*, **10** (suppl. 1): 114–17.

To, L.B., Dyson, P.G. & Juttner, C.A. (1986). Cell-dose effect in circulating stem cell autografting. *Lancet*, **ii**: 404–5 (letter).

To, L.B., Haylock, D.N., Dyson, P.G., Thorp, D., Roberts, M. & Juttner, C.A. (1990). An unusual pattern of haemopoietic reconstitution in patients with acute myeloid leukaemia transplanted with autologous recovery phase peripheral blood. *Bone Marrow Transplant.*, **6**: 109–14.

To, L.B., Haylock, D.N., Kimber, R.J. & Juttner, C.A. (1984). High levels of circulating haemopoietic stem cells in very early remission from acute non-lymphoblastic leukaemia and their collection and cryopreservation. *Br. J. Haematol.*, **58**: 399–410.

To, L.B. & Juttner, C.A. (1987). Peripheral blood stem cell autografting – a new therapeutic option for ANLL? (Annotation) *Br. J. Haematol.*, **66**: 285–289.

To, L.B., Russell, J., Moore, S. & Juttner, C.A. (1987). Residual leukaemia cannot be detected in very early remission peripheral blood stem cell collections in acute non-lymphoblastic leukaemia. *Leuk. Res.*, **11**: 327–330.

10

Blood stem cell transplants in chronic myelogenous leukemia

C. HOYLE AND J.M. GOLDMAN

Introduction

Chronic myelogenous leukemia cannot at present be cured by conventional chemotherapy. Patients in chronic phase have been treated with high doses of cytotoxic drugs but there is little evidence that this prolongs life. With interferon therapy about 70% of patients will achieve a complete hematologic response and 20–40% will achieve some degree of cytogenetic reversion, but even the small minority of patients who achieve sustained cytogenetic remission continue to harbor evidence of the disease at the molecular level. The issue of whether interferon (IFN) prolongs life for perhaps some patients is not yet resolved. Allogeneic bone marrow transplant probably cures most patients who survive the procedure but its use is generally limited to patients under the age of 55 years who are fortunate enough to have HLA-identical siblings. Thus other methods of treating chronic myelogenous leukemia still warrant study. Autografting with blood- or marrow-derived stem cells may lead to sustained Philadelphia (Ph) chromosome negativity in some patients but might delay the onset of transformation and thereby prolong life even in patients who do not achieve Ph chromosome negativity. We review here the rationale for autografting with blood-derived stem cells, the techniques employed and the clinical results.

Theoretical considerations

There is ample evidence that some, if not all, patients with untreated chronic myelogenous leukemia have residual normal hematopoietic stem cells which can in certain circumstances re-establish Ph-negativity (reviewed

117

in Goldman 1991, 1992). Ph-negative hematopoiesis that is usually partial and short-lived can be induced by high dose chemotherapy or by treatment with IFN-α. Perhaps 50% of patients autografted as treatment for acute phase have transient Ph-negative hematopoiesis (Haines *et al.*, 1984). Various laboratory approaches provide further support for this view. For example, Ph-negative progenitor cells can survive in long-term bone marrow culture (Coulombel *et al.*, 1983). Fluorescence-activated cell sorter (FACS) analysis of marrow cells from chronic myelogenous leukemia patients shows that Ph-negative stem cells are found in the $CD34^+/DR^-$ fractions (Verfaillie *et al.*, 1992) and this may be true also for blood cells (De Fabritiis *et al.*, 1993). One recent study showed that a nearly pure population of $CD34^+$ cells with Thy-1 surface marker from which lineage-committed cells had been removed (i.e. $CD34^+/Thy-1^+/lin^-$) was entirely Ph-negative and also negative for BCR/ABL mRNA when studied by the polymerase chain reaction (PCR) (Baum *et al.*, 1992).

It seems probable that Ph-negative progenitors are present in the blood. In the Hammersmith series, 10 of 19 patients autografted with blood stem cells had at least some Ph-chromosome negative marrow metaphases within the first year after autografting. One presumes that engraftment initially results from proliferation of stem cells present in the autografted blood cells but later hematopoiesis may be derived either from transfused stem cells or from 'endogenous' bone marrow cells, or from both. It is possible that blood stem cells differ from marrow-derived stem cells in having a 'limited replicative capacity' (Brito-Babapulle *et al.*, 1989). It is difficult to know whether early engraftment with partially Ph-negative hematopoiesis confers any long-term benefit. Patients in the Hammersmith series who had Ph-negative metaphases detected in the bone marrow within 1 year of autografting survived longer than those who recovered with exclusively Ph-positive hematopoiesis (Fig. 10.1) but the difference is not significant. If early engraftment with Ph-negative stem cells were clinically useful, it would be logical to attempt to mobilize Ph-negative stem cells into the blood before collection by leukapheresis (see below).

How should one collect blood stem cells?

In theory the number of 'normal' stem cells should be greatest before the patient is treated. Alkylating agents such as busulfan are likely to damage the normal stem compartment as much or more than they damage leukemic stem cells and they may predispose to clonal evolution. Thus it would seem appropriate to collect and cryopreserve nucleated cells blood or marrow

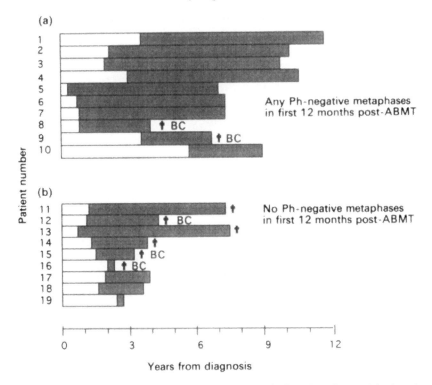

Fig. 10.1. Diagram showing survival from diagnosis for 19 patients with chronic myelogenous leukemia in chronic phase autografted at the Hammersmith Hospital (1984–91). Twenty consecutive patients were autografted in chronic phase. One failed to engraft and is excluded from this analysis. The 19 patients are divided according to whether they had at least some Ph-negative marrow metaphases detectable in the marrow during the first 12 months postautografting (*a*) or only Ph-positive metaphases (*b*). The time of autografting is indicated by the transition from open bar to shaded bar for each patient. ✝ Death. BC, blast crisis. Patient no. 11 committed suicide and patient no. 13 died from hepatitis B infection. ABMT, autologous bone marrow transplant.

cells from all newly diagnosed patients (Goldman *et al.*, 1978; Norman *et al.*, 1981). Such collected nucleated cells will perforce be a mixture of normal and leukemia cells.

It is logical to attempt to collect stem cells from a patient in whom Ph-negativity has been induced by appropriate treatment. The Italian Cooperative Group has autografted a number of patients with marrow cells collected after the patient was treated for varying periods with IFN-α (Baccarani, 1993), but not all patients were Ph-negative at the time of marrow collection. Collection of stem cells from the blood of such patients has not been attempted but might be facilitated by administration of hematopoietic growth factors, such as granulocyte colony-stimulating factor (G-CSF) or granulocyte/macrophage CSF (GM-CSF) (Gianni *et al.*, 1989). The Swedish Cooperative group has autografted patients with marrow collected after intensive chemotherapy (Simonsson *et al.*, 1992). The majority of patients so treated are in continuing cytogenetic remission.

Korbling *et al.* (1981) in Baltimore collected blood stem cells from chronic myelogenous leukemia patients after high dose chemotherapy. These cells were used to autograft the patient in subsequent transformation. The resulting hematopoiesis was entirely Ph-negative. The Genoa group has extended use of this approach (Carella *et al.*, 1991, 1992). They treated a series of chronic myelogenous leukemia patients by chemotherapy and autografting with predominantly Ph-negative blood stem cells collected after high dose chemotherapy for transformation. Some patients were restored to durable Ph-negativity but all eventually died in transformation.

Perhaps the most attractive approach is to develop a method that selectively mobilizes Ph-negative stem cells into the blood. This might be achievable by administering to the patient hematopoietic growth factors such as G-CSF, IL-3, stem cell factor or an appropriate combination of these. There is no information on whether such selectivity can in fact be achieved but G-CSF has stimulated hematopoiesis of donor origin in one Ph-negative patient with leukopenia after allografting (Giralt *et al.*, 1991).

How to condition the patient

It is important to decide the objective of cytoreductive therapy before autografting for patients with chronic myelogenous leukemia in chronic phase. If the intention is to eradicate a maximal number of leukemia stem cells, as is presumably the case prior to allogeneic bone marrow transplants, it seems reasonable to use a chemoradiotherapy schedule known to be effective in allografting, such as cyclophosphamide and total body irradiation. It is worth noting parenthetically that even this schedule does not totally eradicate chronic myelogenous leukemia cells, as attested by the high relapse rate following allografting with T cell depleted donor marrow.

The alternative would be to argue that removal of leukemia stem cells from the harvested blood (or marrow) *in vitro* is unlikely to be totally effective and consequently eradication of chronic myelogenous leukemia from the patient need not necessarily be 'total'. This provides a rationale for less intensive (and presumably less toxic) treatment for the patient. In the past, we at the Hammersmith Hospital used high dose busulfan plus

Table 10.1. *Evolution of approach to the use of cytotoxic drugs (and radiotherapy) for cytoreduction prior to autografting for patients with chronic myelogenous leukemia in complete remission (Hammersmith Hospital, 1984–92)*

Year	Cytoreductive therapy
1984	Cyclophosphamide 60 mg/kg × twice
	Total body irradiation 2 Gy for 6 doses
1985–88	Busulfan 4 mg/m^2 daily for 4 days
	Melphalan 60 mg/m^2 × once
1989–90	Busulfan 4 mg/kg daily for 4 days
	Cyclophosphamide 60 mg/kg × twice
1991–92	Busulfan 4 mg/kg daily for 4 days

melphalan or cyclosphosphamide, now we currently use only busulfan (16 mg/kg) divided over 4 consecutive days (Table 10.1). We have detected no difference in survival in the patients treated with the different regimens.

Blood cell purging *in vitro*

There are a number of possible approaches for manipulation of peripheral blood cells after collection that could theoretically favor marrow reconstitution with Ph-negative stem cells (Table 10.2). Some of these, e.g. incubation with cytotoxic drugs (Degliantoni *et al.*, 1985) and short-term culture in liquid media (Barnett *et al.*, 1989, 1990), have already been tested with chronic myelogenous leukemia marrow cells but one cannot say whether all such methods would be applicable to blood-derived stem cells. The Vancouver group showed that long-term culture initiating cells (LTC-IC) from chronic myelogenous leukemia patients differ from their normal counterparts in a number of ways: they are larger, have higher levels of DR antigen, are brighter when stained by rhodamine and are more sensitive to killing by 4-hydroperoxycyclophosphamide (Udomsakdi *et al.*, 1991). One might speculate therefore that removal of DR positive cells might leave viable CD34$^+$/DR$^-$ cells including Ph-negative LTC-IC which could be used for autografting. One possible problem with this approach is the probability that many of the CD34$^+$/DR$^-$ cells are not in cycle and those that are may produce useful engraftment only after 6–8 weeks.

Removal of chronic myelogenous leukemia progenitors could also be achieved by 'panning', which exploits the aberrant adhesive properties of

Table 10.2. *Approaches to manipulating blood stem cells in vitro to favor reconstitution with Ph-negative hematopoiesis*

Treatment
  Cytotoxic drugs: e.g. mafosfamide, 4HC
  Cytokines: e.g. IL-2, TGF-β
  Cytotoxic drugs plus cytokines: e.g. mafosfamide + MIP-1α
  Monoclonal antibodies
  LAK cells or T cell clones
  BCR/ABL specific antisense oligonucleotides
Short-term incubation (e.g. 10 days)
  Unmodified
  With alpha or gamma interferon
Stem cell selection
  Positive e.g. $CD34^+$, DR^-, $CD38^-$
  Negative
Differential adherence of progenitor cells

MIP-1α, macrophage inflammatory factor 1-α or stem cell inhibitor (Dunlop *et al.*, 1992).

chronic myelogenous leukemia cells. Gordon *et al.* (1987) showed that chronic myelogenous leukemia progenitors adhered less well to a stromal monolayer cultured in the presence of steroids than do comparable normal cells; Verfaillie *et al.* (1992) also demonstrated that chronic myelogenous leukemia cells showed increased binding to laminin and collagen type IV. It would be difficult to use stromal cells for panning on a large scale but technically feasible to use collagen or laminin. It is also possible that small peptides that mimic the binding sites of these molecules could be manufactured cheaply and used to coat flasks suitable for panning. The abnormal adhesive properties of chronic myelogenous leukemia cells could be the reason for their death in the long-term marrow culture systems where they would lack stromal cell contact and maintenance by relevant cytokines.

Incubation of target cells with specific antisense oligonucleotides can suppress their proliferation. Calabretta and colleagues have reported that BCR/ABL specific antisense oligomers will inhibit the proliferation of progenitor cells derived from patients with chronic myelogenous leukemia in transformation (Szczylik *et al.*, 1991). They have also shown that similar oligomers can delay manifestations of leukemia in a mouse-model system in which SCID mice are injected first with BV173 cells (a continuous cell line derived from a patient with chronic myelogenous leukemia in lymphoid transformation) and later with specific antisense sequences (T. Skorski *et al.*, unpublished data). These provocative preclinical observations suggest specific antisense oligomers might be useful for purging chronic myelogenous leukemia blood or marrow cells *in vitro*.

How to assess results

Although there are now a number of published series suggesting that patients with chronic myelogenous leukemia can be autografted with blood- or marrow-derived stem cells and that Ph-negativity can be achieved in some cases, one can draw no firm conclusions about possible benefit for the patient – the ultimate and probably only important criterion being survival. If the majority of an unselected cohort of patients were restored to durable Ph-negativity by autografting, as seems to be the case after allogeneic bone marrow transplants, one might assume that survival had been prolonged and some patients perhaps cured. This has not yet been achieved.

It is likely that various pilot studies designed to achieve durable Ph-negative hematopoiesis in all patients will have to be tested for the next few years. Once a reliable protocol has been identified, carefully controlled studies must be undertaken. The duration of survival for autografted patients must be compared with survival for conventionally treated patients, measured both from the date of diagnosis and from the date of the autograft. We are not yet at the stage where such studies can usefully be implemented.

Recent clinical results

Autografting in transformation

Early clinical studies in Seattle and elsewhere showed that patients with chronic myelogenous leukemia in transformation treated with high dose chemotherapy and marrow autografts would recover chronic phase hematopoiesis (Buckner *et al.*, 1978; Lemmonier *et al.*, 1984). The Hammersmith group showed that the same results could be achieved with patients autografted with blood-derived stem cells (Goldman *et al.*, 1980; Haines *et al.*, 1984). The actual prolongation of life was not, however, sufficiently impressive to justify continuation of this programme.

The group in Genoa has recently reported results of treating 28 patients in blastic transformation by autografting with blood stem cells collected after high dose chemotherapy (idarubicin, cytosine arabinoside and etoposide) (Carella *et al.*, 1992). Eight of these patients achieved Ph-negative hematopoiesis, which was usually short lived. The Bordeaux group has reported results of chemotherapy or chemoradiotherapy followed by autografting in 47 patients with chronic myelogenous leukemia in advanced phases (Reiffers *et al.*, 1986, 1991). Patients received either a single autograft, double autografting or double autografting followed by 'maintenance' with recombinant IFN-α. The median duration of second chronic phase in these three patient groups was 3, 10 and 18 months, respectively. These results are reasonably encouraging in the management of chronic myelogenous leukemia at a phase where other treatment has little or nothing to offer.

Autografting in chronic phase

The Hammersmith group has now used blood-derived stem cells to autograft a total of 20 patients with chronic myelogenous leukemia in chronic phase (Fig. 10.1) (Brito-Babapulle *et al.*, 1989; Hughes *et al.*, 1991). The median survival from autografting is significantly longer than might have been presumed for a comparable group of patients treated by conventional approaches but it is not possible to draw firm conclusions. It is interesting to note that one patient remains Ph-negative for 8 years after autografting (Brito-Babapulle *et al.*, 1987) and a second patient is (80%) Ph-negative at 7 years.

The group in Uppsala autografted ten patients who had achieved Ph-negativity after chemotherapy (Simonsson *et al.*, 1992, see above). All ten patients survive with continuing Ph-negative hematopoiesis. The Genoa group has autografted eight patients with chronic myelogenous leukemia in chronic phase using Ph-negative stem cells collected after 'priming' with high dose chemotherapy (Carella *et al.*, 1992). Six patients recovered with Ph-negative hematopoiesis which was maintained for some months postautografting. Five of these patients were studied for evidence of leukemia using both cytogenetics and polymerase chain reaction.

Future prospects

The value of autografting for chronic myelogenous leukemia remains speculative. If the techniques of allogeneic bone marrow transplants improve substantially within the next few years, such that one can safely transplant older patients and those lacking HLA-identical siblings, autografting will have little role. Conversely, if graft-versus-host disease and opportunistic infections remain major complicating factors, any approach to the management of chronic myelogenous leukemia that offered the prospect of definite prolongation of life, without necessarily cure, would be an important option, especially for the older patient.

References

Baccarani, M. (1993). Chronic myelogenous leukemia: biology and therapy. In *Leukemia*, ed. R.P. Gale, G. Grosveld, E. Canaani & J.M. Goldman. *Leukemia*, **7**: 653–8.

Barnett, M.J., Eaves, C.J., Phillips, G.L. *et al.* (1989). Successful autografting in chronic myeloid leukemia after maintenance of marrow in culture. *Bone Marrow Transplant.*, **4**: 345–51.

Barnett, M.J., Eaves, C.J., Phillips, G.L. *et al.* (1990). Autografting in chronic myeloid leukemia (CML) with cultured marrow: consistent restoration of Philadelphia chromosome (Ph')-negative hematopoiesis in patients selected by prior assessment of their marrow in vitro. *Blood*, **76** (suppl. 1): 526a (abstract no. 2096).

Baum, C.M., Weissman, I.L., Tsukamoto, A.S., Buckle, A.M. & Peault, B. (1992). Isolation of a candidate human hematopoietic stem cell population. *Proc. Natl. Acad. Sci. USA*, **89**: 2804–8.

Brito-Babapulle, F., Apperley, J.F., Rassool, F., Guo, A-P., Dowding, C. & Goldman, J.M. (1987). Complete remission after autografting for chronic myeloid leukemia. *Leuk. Res.*, **11**: 1115–17.

Brito-Babapulle, F., Bowcock, S.J., Marcus, R.E. *et al.* (1989). Autografting for patients with chronic myeloid leukaemia in chronic phase: peripheral blood stem cells may have a finite capacity for maintaining haemopoiesis. *Br. J. Haematol.*, **73**: 76–81.

Buckner, C.D., Stewart, P., Clift, R.A. *et al.* (1978). Treatment of blastic transformation of chronic granulocytic leukemia by chemotherapy, total body irradiation and infusion of cryopreserved autologous marrow. *Exp. Hematol.*, **6**: 96–109.

Carella, A., Gaozza, E., Raffo, M.R. *et al.* (1991). Therapy of acute phase chronic myelogenous leukemia with intensive chemotherapy, blood cell autograft and cyclosporine A. *Leukemia*, **5**: 517–21.

Carella, A.M., Pollicardo, N., Raffo, M.R. *et al.* (1992). Intensive conventional chemotherapy can lead to a precocious overshoot of cytogenetically normal blood stem cells (BSC) in chronic myeloid leukemia and acute lymphoblastic leukemia. *Leukemia*, **6** (suppl. 4): 120–3.

Coulombel, L., Kalousek, D.K., Eaves, C.J., Gupta, C.M. & Eaves, A.C. (1983). Long term marrow culture reveals chromosomally normal hematopoietic progenitor cells in patients with Philadelphia chromosome positive chronic myelogenous leukemia. *N. Engl. J. Med.*, **306**: 1493–8.

De Fabritiis, P., Dowding, D., Bungey, J., Chase, A., Angus, G., Szydlo, R. & Goldman, J.M. Phenotypic characterization of normal and CML CD34-positive cells: only the most primitive CML precursors include Ph-neg cells. *Leukemia Lymphoma* (in press).

Degliantoni, G., Mangoni, L. & Rizzoli, V. (1985). In vitro restoration of polyclonal hematopoiesis in chronic myelogenous leukemia after in vitro treatment with 4-hydroperoxy-cyclophosphamide. *Blood*, **65**: 753–7.

Dunlop, D.J., Wright, E.G., Lorimore, S. *et al.* (1992). Demonstration of stem cell inhibition and myeloprotective effects of SCI/rhMIP1α in vivo. *Blood*, **79**: 2221–5.

Gianni, A.M., Siena, S., Bregni, M. *et al.* (1989). Granulocyte-macrophage CSF to harvest circulate haemopoietic stem cells for autotransplant. *Lancet*, **ii**: 581–4.

Giralt, S., Kantarjian, H., Shahim, S., Cork, A., Fisher, H. & Champlin, R. (1991). Reinduction of durable remission and trilineage response to G-CSF treatment for Ph(−) CML relapsing after allogeneic bone marrow transplant. *Blood*, **78** (suppl 1): 503a (abstract no. 2003).

Goldman, J.M. (1991). Use of autologous stem cells in support of intensive treatment of chronic myelogenous leukemia. In *Chronic Myelogenous Leukemia – Molecular Approaches to Research and Therapy*, ed. A.B. Deisseroth & R.B. Arlinghaus, pp. 455–67. Marcel Dekker Inc, New York.

Goldman, J.M. (1992). Autografting for chronic myeloid leukaemia – palliation, cure or nothing? *Leukemia Lymphoma*, **7**: 51–4.

Goldman, J.M., Johnson, S.A., Islam, A., Catovsky, D. & Galton, D.A.G. (1980). Haematological reconstitution after autografting for chronic granulocytic leukaemia in transformation: the influence of previous splenectomy. *Br. J. Haematol.*, **45**: 223–31.

Goldman, J.M., Th'ng, K.H., Park, D.S., Spiers, A.S.D., Lowenthal, R.M. & Ruutu, T. (1978). Collection, cryopreservation and subsequent viability of haemopoietic stem cells intended for treatment of chronic granulocytic leukaemia in transformation. *Br. J. Haematol.*, **40**: 185–95.

Gordon, M.Y., Dowding, C.R., Riley, G.P., Goldman, J.M. & Greaves, M.F. (1987). Disordered regulation of primitive haemopoietic progenitor cells in chronic myeloid leukaemia is associated with altered interactions with marrow stroma. *Nature*, **328**: 342–4.

Haines, M.E., Goldman, J.M., Worsley, A.M. *et al.* (1984). Chemotherapy and autografting for patients with chronic granulocytic leukaemia in transformation: probable prolongation of life for some patients. *Br. J. Haematol.*, **58**: 711–22.

Hughes, T.P., Brito-Babapulle, F., Tollit, D., Martiat, P., Bowcock, S. & Goldman, J.M. (1991). Induction of Philadelphia-negative hemopoiesis and prolongation of chronic phase in patients with chronic myeloid leukemia treated with high dose chemotherapy and transfusion of peripheral blood stem cells. In *Autologous Bone Marrow Transplantation*, ed. K.A. Dicke, J.O. Armitage, & E. Dicke Evinger, pp. 219–28. University of Nebraska Medical Centre, Omaha.

Korbling, M., Burke, P., Braine, H. *et al.* (1981). Successful engraftment of blood-derived normal hemopoietic stem cells in chronic myelogenous leukemia. *Exp. Hematol.*, **9**: 684–90.

Lemmonier, M.P., Gorin, N.C. & Laporte, J.P. (1984). Autologous marrow transplantation for patients with chronic myelogenous leukemia in accelerated or blastic phase: report of 14 cases. *Exp. Hematol.*, **14**: 654–8.

Norman, J.E., Shepherd, K.M., Dale, B.M. & Sage, R.E. (1981). Collection and cryopreservation of peripheral blood progenitor cells in chronic granulocytic leukaemia–a comparison of treated and untreated patients. *Pathology*, **13**: 609–14.

Reiffers, J., Gorin, N.C., Michallet, M., Maraninchi, D. & Herve, P. (1986). Autografting for chronic granulocytic leukemia in transformation. *J. Natl. Cancer Inst.*, **76**: 1307–11.

Reiffers, J., Trouette, R., Marit, G. *et al.* (1991). Autologous blood stem cell transplantation for chronic granulocytic leukaemia in transformation: a report of 47 cases. *Br. J. Haematol.*, **77**: 339–45.

Szczylik, C., Skorski, T., Nicholaides, N.C. *et al.* (1991). Selective inhibition of leukemia cell proliferation by BCR-ABL antisense oligonucleotides. *Science*, **253**: 562–5.

Simonsson, B., Oberg, G., Bjoreman, M. *et al.* (1992). Intensive treatment in order to minimize the Ph-positive clone in chronic myelogenic leukemia. *Leukemia Lymphoma*, **7**: 55–7.

Udomsakdi, C., Eaves, C.J., Lansdorp, P.M. & Eaves, A.C. (1991). Unique characteristics of primitive neoplastic cells from patients with chronic myeloid leukemia assessed using the long-term culture initiating cells assay. *Blood*, **78** (suppl. 1): 29a (abstract 107).

Verfaillie, C.M., McCarthy, J.B., Miller, W.J. & McGlave, P.B. (1992). Abnormal trafficking of malignant bone marrow progenitors in CML can be explained by their decreased adhesion to stroma and fibronectin but increased adhesion to the basement membrane components laminin and collagen type IV. *Blood*, **78** (suppl. 1): 172a (abstract 680).

11

Blood stem cell transplants in lymphomas
A. KESSINGER AND J.O. ARMITAGE

Introduction

Lymphoma, more than any other malignancy, has been treated with high dose therapy and autologous bone marrow transplants (Bortin *et al.*, 1992). Autologous blood-derived stem cell transplants have been used as a trustworthy alternative to autologous bone marrow transplants for patients whose bone marrows were unsuitable for autografting. Investigators have considered autologous bone marrow unfit when it contained malignant cells that were detectable by light microscopy at the time of, or at any time prior to, stem cell harvesting. Marrow has also been considered unsatisfactory when it was found to be hypocellular in traditional harvest sites, usually as a result of prior chemotherapy or pelvic irradiation (Kessinger *et al.*, 1989; Korbling *et al.*, 1990). In addition, there have been a few anecdotal situations reported where patients eligible for potentially curative marrow ablative therapy could not have been treated without the availability of an alternate source of autologous hematopoietic stem cells. In one instance, a patient had blood stem cells collected after a recently collected autologous bone marrow specimen was inadvertently ruined during attempted cryopreservation, and speedy administration of high dose therapy was considered essential for the patient. The bone marrow collection had required aspirations from an extensive portion of the harvestable sites, and immediate recollection was judged to be impossible (Kessinger *et al.*, 1989). In another instance, a patient with relapsed lymphoma who had bones so dense that marrow aspiration was impossible even while the patient was under general anesthesia, received high dose therapy and blood stem cell transplant (Kessinger *et al.*, 1992). Patients with metastatic malignancy involving the pelvic bone, but not the bone marrow, have had blood stem cell transplants rather than autologous bone marrow transplants because of the concern that harvesting marrow through cancerous bone might result in contamination of the autograft product with malignant cells (Kessinger *et al.*, 1992). A blood stem cell transplant has also been used for a patient whose obesity precluded bone marrow procurement.

Some patients with relapsed lymphomas have had blood stem cell transplants rather than autologous bone marrow transplants after high dose therapy because recovery of hematopoiesis was expected to be more rapid (Gianni *et al.*, 1989; Kotasek *et al.*, 1992). This result can be anticipated only if the number of stem cells in the blood stream is deliberately expanded during the collection process.

The number of patients reported in the literature who have received high dose therapy and blood stem cell transplants for relapsed lymphoma now has surpassed 200. Some had been observed for only a short interval at the time they were described in the literature, but others were reported after a sufficient length of time had elapsed to demonstrate that long-term disease-free survival can result from this therapeutic approach.

Hodgkin's disease

At least 123 relapsed Hodgkin's disease patients treated with high dose therapy and blood stem cell transplants have been reported in the literature (Lasky *et al.*, 1989; Reiffers *et al.*, 1989; Zander *et al.*, 1989; Williams *et al.*, 1990; Haas *et al.*, 1992; Kessinger *et al.*, 1992). The vast majority of these patients received blood stem cell transplants because they had an underlying marrow abnormality that precluded an autologous bone marrow transplant. Several of the reports included a small number of patients with brief follow-up, but two larger series had sufficient follow-up reported to permit some initial insight into the potential efficacy of this therapeutic approach.

Haas *et al.* (1992) described 28 Hodgkin's disease patients whose lymphoma had relapsed following primary combination chemotherapy. In addition, these patients had also received prior radiation therapy to traditional harvest sites, which made collection of adequate marrow for autografting impossible. Following relapse but prior to high dose therapy and blood stem cell transplants they were all treated with salvage chemotherapy and demonstrated a tumor response (i.e. had a sensitive relapse). The high dose chemotherapy consisted of cyclophosphamide (6–6.8 g/m²), carmustine (600–800 mg/m²) and etoposide (1000–1600 mg/m²). Four patients experienced a toxic death after transplant. Six further patients had disease relapse or progression 1–7 months after the transplant. The remaining 18 patients were reported to be free from disease at a median of 17 months (range 2–57 months) after blood stem cell transplant. These results suggest that long-term event-free survival is possible for some patients with relapsed Hodgkin's disease that remained responsive to conventional doses of chemotherapy when treated with high dose therapy and blood stem cell transplants.

Another published series of Hodgkin's disease patients treated with high dose therapy and blood stem cell transplants (Kessinger *et al.*, 1992) was updated for this review. Ninety-two consecutive adult patients with relapsed or refractory Hodgkin's disease were treated. All patients had a bone marrow abnormality that precluded an autologous bone marrow transplant. Of the patients studied, not all were in sensitive relapse. The high dose therapy consisted of cyclophosphamide, etoposide and carmustine for all but one patient. Four patients had a toxic death after blood stem cell transplant. Of 29 patients, 26 have died of progressive disease, 1 from coccidiomycosis and 1 from idiopathic thrombocytopenic purpura, also there was 1 suicide. Thirty-seven patients remained event-free (survival without disease progression or the appearance of a second primary malignancy) 41–1747 days (median 739 days) after transplant. Some of these event-free survivors, including the patient who was followed for the longest period of time, had histopathologic proof of bone marrow metastases at the time of high dose therapy and blood stem cell transplants. The actuarial event-free survival for all 92 patients 58 months after transplant was 23%. While this series of patients has demonstrated that long-term event-free survival is possible for patients who have relapsed Hodgkin's disease and are treated with high dose therapy and blood stem cell transplants, the follow-up has not been extended sufficiently to establish the curative potential of this approach.

Non-Hodginson's lymphoma

Patients with low, intermediate and high grade non-Hodginson's lymphomas have been treated with high dose therapy and blood stem cell transplants. Most of the patients reported thus far have relapsed or have refractory lymphoma at the time of the transplant, but some patients with poor risk disease have received high dose therapy as consolidation after achieving a complete remission with conventional therapeutic approaches (Korbling *et al.*, 1986; Takaue *et al.*, 1991; Majolino *et al.*, 1992). In addition, an occasional patient was treated with high dose therapy and blood stem cell transplant as initial therapy (Kotasek *et al.*, 1992). Some patients who received high dose therapy were rescued with autologous blood stem cells because they had marrow metastases or marrow hypocellularity and others because their blood stem cells were mobilized during the collections and a rapid hematopoietic recovery was anticipated.

At least 91 non-Hodginson's lymphoma patients treated with high dose therapy and blood stem cell transplants have been reported, and two series of such patients have recently been analyzed for long-term outcome. Kotasek *et al.* (1992) reviewed the clinical course of 16 poor risk patients who had mostly intermediate and high grade non-Hodginson's lymphoma. The patients all received high dose BCNU, etoposide, cytarabine and melphalan followed by mobilized blood stem cell transplants. At the time the high dose therapy was administered, ten patients were in complete remission, three patients were in partial remission and two patients were experiencing progressive disease. At a median follow-up of 528 days (range 77–840 days) after blood stem cell transplant, six patients were dead, three were alive with progressive disease, and seven were surviving free of disease 77–734 days after transplant, although two of these patients may have relapsed after transplant and achieved another complete remission with additional therapy.

A larger series of 48 patients with intermediate and high grade non-Hodginson's lymphoma, who were treated with high dose therapy and blood stem cell transplants, has been described (Kessinger & Armitage, 1992). All patients had either relapsed or refractory disease at the time of blood stem cell collection, and all patients had bone marrow that was considered unsuitable for autografting, most often as a result of hypocellularity or evidence of metastatic disease in the marrow. Mobilization methods were not used during blood stem cell harvesting for any of the patients. Three different high dose therapy regimens were utilized and the specific therapy was assigned according to the histologic subtype as well as the demonstrated responsiveness of the lymphoma being treated to chemotherapy. Thirteen patients received cyclophosphamide and total body irradiation, 19 patients received BCNU, etoposide, cyclophosphamide and cytarabine, and 15 patients received BCNU, etoposide, cyclophosphamide and hydroxyurea. Twenty-one patients (44%) achieved a complete remission after blood stem cell transplants. The actuarial event-free survival for all 48 patients at 57 months was 28%. The possibility of cure for some of these patients was suggested by the shape of the survival curve (rapid early fall off and then a plateau), and by the length of event-free survival for at least some of the patients with an otherwise aggressive disease.

Another series of patients with nontransformed low grade non-Hodginson's lymphoma has been treated with high dose therapy and blood stem cell transplants (Bierman *et al.*, 1992). An update of that series revealed that 30 patients have been treated. They all had experienced disease progression after at least one trial of chemotherapy, and all had bone marrow abnormalities that made autologous bone marrow transplants untenable. If the patients had not received radiation therapy earlier in their disease course (24 patients), they were treated with cyclophosphamide and total body irradiation. Six patients who were ineligible for total body irradiation received BCNU, etoposide, cyclophosphamide and cytarabine as the high dose therapy. Sixty-three per cent of the patients achieved a complete response. The actuarial event-free survival 40 months after blood stem cell transplant was 39%. Follow-up for this group of patients is still too short to ascertain whether cures can result for patients with low grade non-Hodginson's lymphoma using this approach.

Conclusion

Less than a decade ago, modern high dose therapy and blood stem cell transplants were first used for the management of Hodgkin's disease and non-Hodginson's lymphoma. Now, more than 200 patients treated with this approach have been reported, and as a result of the increased numbers of patients treated and the longer periods of observation, the value of the therapy is becoming clearer. About 30% of patients with persistent Hodgkin's disease have experienced long-term event-free survival following high dose therapy and autologous bone marrow transplants (Kessinger *et al.*, 1990), and this result apparently can also be achieved with high dose therapy and blood stem cell transplants.

While follow-up is still too brief to ascertain the curative potential of high dose therapy and blood stem cell or autologous bone marrow transplants for low grade non-Hodginson's lymphoma, clearly long-term survival has resulted for a number of patients transplanted with either marrow or blood-derived stem cells. High dose therapy and autologous bone marrow transplants have produced long-term survival and probable cure for approximately 30% of patients with relapsed intermediate and high grade non-Hodginson's lymphoma (Kessinger *et al.*, 1990), and the available data suggest that very similar results can be expected for similar patients treated with high dose therapy and blood stem cell transplants.

References

Bierman, P., Vose, J., Armitage, J. & Kessinger, A. (1992). High-dose therapy followed by autologous hematopoietic rescue for follicular low grade non-Hodgkin's lymphoma (NHL). *Proc. Am. Soc. Clin. Oncol.*, **11**: 1074.

Bortin, M.M., Horowitz, M.M. & Rimm, A.A. (1992). Increasing utilization of allogeneic bone marrow transplantation. Results of the 1988–1990 survey. *Ann. Intern. Med.*, **116**: 505–12.

Gianni, A.M., Siena, S., Bregni, M. *et al.* (1989). Granulocyte-macrophage colony-stimulating factor to harvest circulating haemopoietic stem cells for autotransplantation. *Lancet*, **ii**: 580–5.

Haas, R., Hohaus, S., Egerer, G., Ogniben, E., Witt, B. & Hunstein, W. (1992). Autologous blood stem cell transplantation in relapsed Hodgkin's disease. *Int. J. Cell Cloning*, **10** (suppl. 1): 138–40.

Kessinger, A. & Armitage, J.O. (1992). Peripheral stem cell transplantation for patients with non-Hodgkin lymphoma. *Int. J. Cell Cloning*, **10** (suppl. 1): 127–8.

Kessinger, A., Armitage, J.O., Smith, D.M., Landmark, J.D., Bierman, P.J. & Weisenburger, D.D. (1989). High-dose therapy and autologous blood stem cell transplantation for patients with lymphoma. *Blood*, **74**: 1260–5.

Kessinger, A., Nademanee, A., Forman, S.J. & Armitage, J.O. (1990). Autologous bone marrow transplantation for Hodgkin's and non-Hodgkin's lymphoma. *Hematol. Oncol. Clin. North Am.*, **4**: 577–87.

Kessinger, A., Vose, J.M., Bierman, P.J. & Armitage, J.O. (1992). High dose cyclophosphamide, etoposide and carmustine and peripheral stem cell transplantation for patients with relapsed Hodgkin disease and bone marrow abnormalities. *Int. J. Cell Cloning*, **10** (suppl. 1): 135–7.

Korbling, M., Dorken, B., Ho, A.D., Pezzutto, A., Hunstein, W. & Fliedner, T.M. (1986). Autologous transplantation of blood-derived hemopoietic stem cells after myeloablative therapy in a patient with Burkitt's lymphoma. *Blood*, **67**: 529–32.

Korbling, M., Holle, R., Haas, R. *et al.* (1990). Autologous blood stem-cell transplantation in patients with advanced Hodgkin's disease and prior radiation to the pelvic site. *J. Clin. Oncol.*, **8**: 978–85.

Kotasek, D., Sage, R.E., Juttner, C.A. & To, L.B. (1992). Autologous transplantation in non-Hodgkin's lymphomas using high dose cyclophosphamide mobilized blood stem cells: the Adelaide experience. *Int. J. Cell Cloning*, **10** (suppl. 1): 129–31.

Lasky, L.C., Hurd, D.D., Smith, J.A. & Haake, R. (1989). Peripheral blood stem cell collection and use in Hodgkin's disease. Comparison with marrow in autologous transplantation. *Transfusion*, **29**: 323–7.

Majolino, I., Quaglietta, A.M., Iacone, A. *et al.* (1992). *Int. J. Cell Cloning*, **10** (suppl. 1): 132–4.

Reiffers, J., Leverger, G., Marit, S. *et al.* (1989). Haematopoietic reconstitution after autologous blood stem cell transplantation. In *Bone Marrow Transplantation Current Controversies*, ed. R.P. Gale & R.E. Champlin, pp. 313–20. Alan R. Liss, New York.

Takaue, Y., Watanabe, T., Hoshi, Y. *et al.* (1991). Effectiveness of high-dose MCNU therapy and hematopoietic stem cell autografts treatment of childhood acute leukemia/lymphoma with high-risk features. *Cancer*, **67**: 1830–7.

Williams, S.F., Bitran, J.D., Richards, P.J. *et al.* (1990). Peripheral blood-derived stem cell collections for use in autologous transplantation after high dose chemotherapy: an alternative approach. *Bone Marrow Transplant.*, **5**: 129–33.

Zander, A.R., Lyding, J., Cockerill, K.J., Askamit, I. & Shepherd, R. (1989). Autologous blood stem cell transplantation. In *Autologous Bone Marrow Transplantation, Proceedings of the Fourth International Symposium*, ed. K.A. Dicke, G. Spitzer, S. Jagannath & M.J. Evinger-Hodges, pp. 713–17. University of Texas M.D. Anderson Cancer Center Press, Houston.

12

Blood stem cell transplants in breast cancer
K.H. ANTMAN

Conventional therapy for breast cancer

Breast cancer currently develops in one of every nine American and northern European women. While less common in Japan, the incidence there is also increasing. Rates for southern Europeans fall between those for American and Japanese women. Relapse rates at 10 years increase proportionally to the number of axillary lymph nodes, from approximately 20% for patients with no positive lymph nodes, 60% for one to three lymph nodes involved and more than 85% for four or more axillary lymph nodes involved. Women with stage 2 disease with more than ten positive lymph nodes and locally advanced or inflammatory breast cancer have a very poor prognosis with conventional therapy. Relapse tends to occur earlier for patients with higher numbers of lymph nodes involved, and some risk of relapse remains for at least 20 years after mastectomy. Prognosis is worse for patients with poorly differentiated tumors, high nuclear grade, greater than a diploid number of chromosomes, high fraction of cells synthesizing DNA (S-phase fraction) and those with extra copies of *Her* 2/ *neu* oncogene.

Women with metastatic breast cancer are essentially incurable with conventional therapy, with a median survival of about 2 years after documentation of metastases (Clark *et al.*, 1987; Mick *et al.*, 1989). The median survival of women with metastatic disease has not changed in the five decades for which statistics are available. While generally sensitive to initial chemotherapy regimens, metastatic breast cancer virtually always progresses with shorter and less complete responses with subsequent regimens. Women with estrogen receptor positive tumors (median 2.3 years), and those who achieve a complete response with conventional dose therapy (median 2.5 years) or who have only small amounts of local disease (median >4 years) have a somewhat better survival (Mick *et al.*, 1989).

Metastatic breast cancer therefore represents a major public health problem, as well as a frightening personal situation for women afflicted with the disease.

Dose intensive therapy in breast cancer

Rationale

In laboratory models of breast cancer and other malignancies, the delivery of the highest possible doses of chemotherapy is essential to achieve curative therapy. Theory, experimental and clinical data suggest that breast cancer recurs despite an initial response to chemotherapy because of resistance to the chemotherapy drugs. In the laboratory, resistance to alkylating agents can often be overcome by using a five to ten fold higher dose. Laboratory models have been reviewed (Frei *et al.*, 1989).

Clinically, some correlation between chemotherapy dose and response is also recognized (Frei & Canellos, 1980). In 1984, Hryniuk & Bush introduced the concept of dose intensity to attempt to quantify dose–response effects using metastatic breast cancer as a model. The dose-intensity methodology has been widely debated (Henderson *et al.*, 1988; Cohen *et al.*, 1990). Given theoretical concerns, a review of randomized clinical trials in which dose intensity is the most important variable seems appropriate. While some of these trials have shown an increased response rate for regimens with greater dose intensity, few trials demonstrate a significantly increased overall survival. In the trial by Tannock *et al.* (1988), randomization resulted in an excess of patients with brief durations between initial diagnosis and relapse on the low dose intensity arm causing the authors to advise caution in the interpretation of the survival advantage observed in their trial. The trial, however, did suggest that the increased response rate also observed was associated with an improved quality of life (Tannock *et al.*, 1988). Carmo-Pereira *et al.* (1987) demonstrated a statistically significant difference in median survival (8 months versus 20 months) for patients receiving two different doses of doxorubicin. These randomized trials suggest that modest increments in dose intensity produce, at best, only modest effects on survival. The general lack of an improvement in survival for the higher dose intensity arms may reflect the relatively minor differences in dose administered, or the lack of any major effect of conventional chemotherapy regimens on median survival in metastatic breast cancer. Mathematical models of breast cancer by Norton

& Day (1991) suggest that because of Gompertzian growth of residual tumor, differences in survival are difficult to document unless a substantial fraction of patients is cured.

Rationale for stem cell support

Escalation of drugs such as cyclophosphamide and doxorubicin result in dose-limiting cardiac toxicity without requiring hematopoietic stem cells (Appelbaum et al., 1976; Herzig et al., 1981, 1987; Elias et al., 1990). Significant escalations of combinations such as CAF (cyclophosphamide, doxorubicin and 5-fluorouracil) or CPE (cyclophosphamide, cisplatin and etoposide) have been possible without stem cell support (Spitzer et al., 1987; Demetri et al., 1991b). Other agents active in breast cancer such as thiotepa or melphalan can be escalated only one to twofold with hematopoietic growth factors but 3–40-fold with autotransplants. For example, the usual dose of thiotepa is 40 mg/m². The maximum tolerated dose with granulocyte colony-stimulating factor (G-CSF) support is 75 mg/m² (Schilder et al., 1991); however 1.0–1.5 gm/m² can be delivered with autotransplant (Herzig et al., 1987; Wolff et al., 1989; Schilder et al., 1990).

Many authors have used autotransplants to ensure prompt marrow recovery after high doses of chemotherapy because the limiting toxicity of higher chemotherapy doses is myelosuppression. Breast cancer is an optimal tumor for studies of the role of high dose therapy based on its sensitivity at conventional chemotherapy doses.

Results of high dose studies

Currently available published trials have now documented that dose-intensive chemotherapy with autotransplantation is an effective treatment for metastatic breast cancer. Several high dose regimens tested in patients with no prior chemotherapy for stage IV disease or responding to conventional dose treatment have resulted in a complete response rate higher than that generally reported with conventional dose treatment. Complete responses have proven relatively durable, whereas partial responses have been brief. A quarter to a half of those achieving complete response have no evidence of progression with follow-up intervals in the range 2–4 years in trials carried out by groups of institutions (Antman et al., 1991, 1992). Patients should be selected carefully. Because of the toxicity (and costs) associated with this treatment, it appears clear at

Table 12.1. *Summary of patient outcome of women treated with high dose cyclophosphamide, thiotepa and carboplatin (CTCb) at the Dana-Farber Cancer Institute*

Number of women transplanted	53	
Toxic deaths	2	4%
Evaluable for response	51	
Complete response or PR[a]	29	57%
(CR save for residual bone scan uptake)		
Without progression	20	39%
Transplanted prior to 19 January 1990 (i.e. 2–4 year follow-up)	30	
Without progression	8	27%

[a]PR is defined as complete response save for residual abnormal bone scan. Once abnormal, bone scans do not again become normal, even if disease responds; CR, complete remission.

present that those with refractory or bulky disease are unlikely to achieve a complete response.

While any treatment-related mortality is to be avoided, metastatic breast cancer is invariably fatal with a median duration of remission of 8 months and a median survival of 1.6 years, therefore some risk is justified. Mortality rates of conventional dose chemotherapy for metastatic disease is in the range 2–4%. Mortality rates for dose-intensive therapy in breast cancers have ranged from 3% to 24% (Antman *et al.*, 1991, 1992). Mortality rates of 50% are acceptable in the setting of allogeneic marrow transplant for second remission acute myeloid leukemia with a cure rate of ~20–30%.

Results of the Dana-Farber Cancer Institute

In the phase II study, CTCb (cyclophosphamide, thiotepa and carboplatin) (Table 12.1) was demonstrated to be an intensification regimen with a low mortality which achieves the goal of delivery of significantly increased doses of agents known to be active at conventional doses in breast cancer (Antman *et al.*, 1992). Profound myelosuppression and some mucositis was considered acceptable but agents with organ toxicity such as doxorubicin or BCNU were avoided in the construction of this transplant regimen (Eder *et al.*, 1990). The duration of partial responses were short, as predicted by modeling experiments and observed studies of marrow transplant in patients with leukemia and lymphoma. The impact of less than two logs of tumor cytotoxicity (i.e. a partial response) is small if tumor growth kinetics are assumed to be Gompertzian (Norton & Day, 1991).

Complete responses (whether achieved after induction or after intensification) appeared to be relatively durable as did responses in patients with only residual positive bone scans and sclerosis on X-ray.

Bone marrow involvement by breast cancer

More than 40% of patients with metastatic breast cancer and about 55% of those with a positive bone scan or metastases evident on bone X-rays have bone marrow involvement detected by conventional studies of bone marrow biopsies, aspirations or clot sections (Ingle *et al.*, 1978; Ellis *et al.*, 1989).

Recent studies designed to detect epithelial cells in histologically normal bone marrow using monoclonal antibodies (Hilkens *et al.*, 1983; Kufe *et al.*, 1984) have suggested that approximately one-third of patients with stage II primary breast cancer have bone marrow micrometastatic involvement (Redding *et al.*, 1983; Cote *et al.*, 1991). The latter investigators have reported that the detection of bone marrow micrometastases is predictive of early relapse, suggesting that these cells are viable and that bone marrow contamination is clinically important.

The importance of either overt or occult bone marrow involvement in the setting of autologous bone marrow transplants is unknown. Tumor cells have been reported by investigators in Nebraska to grow in long-term cultures of marrow from breast cancer patients with histologically normal diagnostic marrow samples (Mann *et al.*, 1986). Growth of tumor cells in tissue culture correlates with breast cancer recurrence (Vaughan *et al.*, 1990). Chemotherapy given prior to bone marrow procurement may reduce or eliminate tumor cells *in vivo* and permit autotransplants with minimal risk of reinoculating the patient with viable autologous malignant cells.

Few if any studies of tumor contamination of blood stem cell products collected either with unperturbed hematopoiesis or mobilized by chemotherapy and hematopoietic growth factors have been published. One suggests decreased contamination using blood stem cells compared with marrow (Sharp *et al.*, 1992). Receptors for GM-CSF and G-CSF, nevertheless, have been found on the surface of several types of malignant cells, and GM-CSF has been reported to be a growth stimulus for cells of a human breast cancer line (Dedhar *et al.*, 1988; Baldwin *et al.*, 1989; Berdel *et al.*, 1989; Avalos *et al.*, 1990). It is theoretically possible that similar modulation of adhesion molecules to the effects of GM-CSF on blood stem cells might occur on breast cancer cells *in vivo*, resulting in significant tumor cell contamination of a blood stem cell product harvested from patients treated with hematopoietic growth factors. This represents an important research question with potentially therapeutic implications.

Cost effectiveness

Concurrent studies of prophylactic antibiotics, colony-stimulating factors and peripheral blood stem cell support may substantially decrease the morbidity and the length of admissions for patients receiving high dose therapy, significantly decreasing the cost. A preliminary analysis of costs based on 3-year data from the Duke program compared with conventional dose therapy on cancer and leukemia group B studies estimates that the current cost of dose intensive therapy per year of life saved is $85000. (The costs of conventional dose therapy and dose intensive therapy were estimated at $31500 and $73300, respectively.) Thus, current costs are 'very high and greater than most but not all acceptable therapies'. If the complete remissions prove to be durable and growth factors and blood progenitor cell support significantly lower the costs, dose-intensive therapy may prove both clinically and cost effective (Hillner *et al.*, 1991).

Hematopoietic stem cells collected from peripheral blood

The concentration of hematopoietic stem cells in the blood is 10–100-fold less than in marrow. There is no clear understanding either of why hematopoietic stem cells circulate peripherally or of their regulation. Stem cells collected from the peripheral blood of laboratory animals by cytopheresis have successfully reconstituted myelopoiesis following marrow lethal treatment (Weiner *et al.*, 1977; Sarpel *et al.*, 1979).

Adequacy and speed of recovery appears related in part to the number of stem cells reinfused. Assays of committed progenitor cells (colony-forming unit granulocyte/macrophage, CFU-GM) have been used as surrogate markers of the presence and quantity of stem cells as there are no assays for the true human stem cells. Approximately 4×10^5 CFU-GM/kg body weight (15–50-fold that required for autologous bone marrow transplants) are apparently sufficient for reliable reconstitution after marrow ablative therapy. The disparity between the number of marrow and blood CFU-GM required may reflect a lower ratio of pluripotent to committed stem cells in peripheral blood or to the few stromal cells transplanted (Bell *et al.*, 1986; To & Juttner, 1987). Five to eight leukapheresis are required for adequate blood stem cell collection in humans with unperturbed hematopoiesis (Goldman *et al.*, 1978; Juttner *et al.*, 1986; Ho *et al.*, 1990; Kessinger *et al.*, 1992).

Kessinger *et al.* (1986) have refined the technical collection of blood stem cells from patients with undisturbed hematopoiesis and documented successful engraftment in 34 breast cancer and Hodgkin's disease patients treated with cyclophosphamide, total body irradiation and cisplatin.

Potential advantages and disadvantages of blood stem cells compared with marrow

Breast cancer contamination of blood stem cell collections has been reported at a lower incidence than of marrow in one report (Sharp *et al.*, 1992). The incidence of contamination remains an important target for further investigation.

The accumulated data to date suggest that blood or marrow stem cells are capable of re-engrafting hematopoiesis at about equivalent rates (To & Juttner, 1987; Siena *et al.*, 1989; Ho *et al.*, 1990; Shea *et al.*, 1990; Elias *et al.*, 1991a,b; Mazanet *et al.*, 1991). Leukapheresis to harvest blood stem cells from the circulation is an outpatient procedure similar to platelet donation. Adequate numbers of stem cells may be collected from patients with hemipelvectomies, tumor involving the pelvic bones, or after pelvic irradiation. One major disadvantage to the routine use of blood stem cells collected without mobilization is the seven to ten leukaphereses required for adequate stem cell collection. The number of collections required strains blood bank and cryopreservation resources and delays therapy.

Methods of increasing CFU-GM yields during leukapheresis

Unsuccessful methods to increase the number of blood stem cells have included dextran, steroids, and endotoxin (Bell *et al.*, 1986; To & Juttner, 1987). Considerable interest has been generated, however, by the observation that blood stem cells can be mobilized into the circulation by intensive chemotherapy (Richman *et al.*, 1976; Lohrmann *et al.*, 1978; Abrams *et al.*, 1981; Ruse-Riol *et al.*, 1984; To *et al.*, 1984; Socinski *et al.*, 1988), hematopoietic growth factor administration (Socinski *et al.*, 1988), or a combination of these two. A consistent feature of these mobilized blood stem cells compared with marrow transplants has been rapid granulocyte reconstitution (8–16 days to $> 500 \times 10^6/l$) possibly resulting from reinfusion

Table 12.2. *Effect of GM-CSF on the number of CFU-GM and BFU-E in the peripheral blood with and without chemotherapy*

Progenitor cell subset	Pre-treatment	Post-GM-CSF alone	Post-GM-CSF with chemotherapy	Post-chemotherapy alone
CFU-GM	36	469	2251	74
BFU-E	68	242	1125	80

Numbers refer to the concentration of progenitor cells in the peripheral blood (i.e. no. of cells/ml of blood).
BFU-E, blood-forming unit-erythropoietic; CFU-GM, colony-forming unit-granulocyte/macrophage; GM-CSF, granulocyte/macrophage colony-stimulating factor.
Source: Socinski *et al.* (1988).

of larger number of committed progenitor cells and equivalent rates of platelet recovery (19–25 days). More rapid hematologic reconstitution would substantially reduce mortality, morbidity and the expense of high dose therapy (Gianni *et al.*, 1989a, b, c; Siena *et al.*, 1989; Ravagnani *et al.*, 1990; Elias *et al.*, 1991a,b; Mazanet *et al.*, 1991).

Effect of GM-CSF on blood stem cells

We have shown that GM-CSF, particularly given during the period of chemotherapy-induced rebound, significantly increased absolute numbers of peripheral blood CFU-GM (median 18-fold, range 2–200-fold) ($p = 0.01$). The concentration of BFU-E (burst forming unit-erythrocyte) in the circulation increased a median of 8-fold. In the marrow, however, bone marrow CFU-GM and BFU-E numbers did not significantly change (Socinski *et al.*, 1988) (Table 12.2).

Numerous other investigators have confirmed these observations of stem cell mobilization into the peripheral blood after administration of GM-CSF, G-CSF (To & Juttner, 1987; Siena *et al.*, 1989; Crouse *et al.*, 1990; Toki *et al.*, 1990; Elias *et al.*, 1991a,b; Mazanet *et al.*, 1991) or IL-3 (Demetri *et al.*, 1991a).

The molecular mechanisms by which hematopoietic growth factors such as GM-CSF or G-CSF mobilize hematopoietic stem cells is unknown but is likely to involve alterations in the presence, quantity, or ligand recognition by adhesion structures on the surface of the stem cells (Griffin *et al.*, 1990).

Our group has observed that 24 women with advanced breast cancer who

Table 12.3. *Conventional-dose 'induction' therapy*

Cycle	1	2	3	4	High dose treatment
Chemotherapy GM-CSF 5 μg/kg days 6–15 continuous infusion	AF[a] M	AF	AF	AF M	CTCb[b]
2 h Leukapheresis (days 15–18) Reinfusion of all blood stem cells collected			↑↑	↑↑	
Marrow harvest as reserve		◇			◇

Blood stem cells reinfused on day 0. ↑↑ = drug delivery. ◇, ◇ = collection and reinfusion of marrow.
[a] A = doxorubicin 25 mg/m^2 on days 3–5, F = 5-fluorouracil 600 mg/m^2 on days 1–5, M = methotrexate 250 mg/m^2 on day 18, with leucovorin rescue.
[b] CTCb = cyclophosphamide, thiotepa, carboplatin (6000, 500, 800 mg/m^2, respectively) over 4 days continuous infusion on days −7 to −3.
GM-CSF, granulocyte/macrophage colony-stimulating factor.

received GM-CSF-mobilized blood stem cells (without marrow) had a significantly shorter time to hematopoietic recovery after high dose cyclophosphamide, thiotepa and carboplatin than 25 historical controls who had received the same high dose combination chemotherapy regimen supported by autologous marrow stem cells. Other groups have combined blood stem cells and marrow (Siena *et al.*, 1989; Mazanet *et al.*, 1991).

Use of hematopoietic growth factors and blood stem cells to reduce toxicities associated with high dose therapy

In randomized clinical studies, G-CSF (Masaoka *et al.*, 1990) and GM-CSF (Philip *et al.*, 1989; Gorin *et al.*, 1990; Link *et al.*, 1990; Michon *et al.*, 1990; Nemunaitis *et al.*, 1991) given after marrow transplant resulted in a modest but statistically significant decreased time to reengraftment, number of infectious complications, days with an absolute neutrophil count (ANC) < 1.0, days with an absolute neutrophil count (ANC) $< 1.0 \times 10^9/l$ and number of hospital days.

A pilot study was designed to determine whether blood stem cells mobilized by GM-CSF during the recovery from cytotoxic chemotherapy can accelerate hematologic recovery following high dose CTCb chemotherapy in patients with advanced breast cancer who had responded to conventional dose 'induction' therapy. The study schema is shown in Table 12.3.

Eligible patients had metastatic breast cancer. Endpoints included the time to unmaintained hematologic recovery and durability of engraftment for each cell lineage. Fifteen patients were entered. One patient died from chronic heart failure during recovery after CTCb high dose therapy. Platelet recovery was incomplete in two patients who required reinfusion of the previously stored backup marrow. A third patient who received radiotherapy to her chest wall after transplant, also received her marrow reinfusion when her disease progressed after high dose therapy and she required additional treatment.

These 15 patients who received blood stem cells were compared with 29 patients treated on the immediately prior study with the same high dose chemotherapy regimen (CTCb) with marrow support alone. Fewer red blood cell and platelet transfusions were required. Days to ANC < $500 \times 10^6/l$, platelets > $20 \times 10^9/l$ and hospital discharge were reduced by a median of 7, 11 and 14 days, respectively. The use of blood stem cells as support for high dose chemotherapy appears to provide durable and rapid engraftment in the majority of cases and is likely to result in lower morbidity and cost for transplantation.

Table 12.4. *Time to re-engraftment for three sequential studies*

	BSC/GM-CSF	BSC alone	Marrow alone
Number of patients with responding breast cancer	9	15	29
Days from reinfusion to:			
Neutrophils $> 500 \times 10^6/l$	11 (10–45)	14 (10–57)	21 (12–51)
Platelets $> 20 \times 10^9/l$	11 (7–28$^+$)	12 (8–134)	24 (7–83)
Hospital days	24 (21–77)	24 (19–34)	32 (21–112)

BSC, blood stem cell; GM-CSF, granulocyte/macrophage colony-stimulating factor.
Source: Elias *et al.* (1991a,b).

In an ongoing follow-up study of the same treatment protocol, GM-CSF was also given after reinfusion of blood stem cells. A summary of the results of time to re-engraftment for the three sequential studies is given in Table 12.4.

Further research is ongoing at the Dana-Farber Cancer Institute in the study of blood stem cell support for breast cancer patients treated with dose-intensive chemotherapy regimens, based on the extremely promising results observed here and at other institutions worldwide (Kessinger *et al.*, 1986; To & Juttner, 1987; Peters *et al.*, 1989; Ho *et al.*, 1990; Shea *et al.*, 1990; Elias *et al.*, 1990; Mazanet *et al.*, 1991).

References

Abrams, R.A., Johnston-Early, A., Cramer, C., Minna, J.D., Cohen, M.H. & Deisseroth, M. (1981). Amplification of circulating granulocyte-monocyte stem cell numbers following chemotherapy in patients with extensive small cell carcinoma of the lung. *Cancer Res.*, **41**: 35–41.

Antman, K., Ayash, L., Elias, A. *et al.* (1992). A phase II study of high dose cyclophosphamide, thiotepa, and carboplatin with autologous marrow support in women with measurable advanced breast cancer responding to standard dose therapy. *J. Clin. Oncol.*, **10**: 102–10.

Antman, K., Bearman, S., Davidson, N. *et al.* (1991). High dose therapy in breast cancer with autologous bone marrow support: current status. In *New Strategies in Bone Marrow Transplantation (new series in Molecular & Cellular Biology)*, ed. R.P. Gale & R.E. Champolan, Alan R. Liss, New York. 423–36.

Appelbaum, F.R., Stauchen, J.A., Graw, R.G. *et al.* (1976). Acute lethal carditis caused by high dose combination chemotherapy: a unique clinical and pathologic indice. *Lancet*, **1**: 58–62.

Avalos, B.R., Gasson, J.C., Hedrat, C. *et al.* (1990). Human granulocyte colony-stimulating factor: biologic activities and receptor characterization on hematopoietic cells and small cell lung cancer cell lines. *Blood*, **75**: 851–7.

Baldwin, G.C., Gasson, J.C., Kaufman, S.E. *et al.* (1989). Nonhematopoietic tumor cells express functional GM-CSF receptors. *Blood*, 73: 1033–7.

Bell, A.J., Hamblin, T.J. & Oscier, D.A. (1986). Circulating stem cell autografts. *Bone Marrow Transplant.*, 1: 103–10.

Berdel, W.E., Danhauser, R.S., Steinhauser, S. & Winton, E.F. (1989). Various human hematopoietic growth factors (interleukin-3, GM-CSF, G-CSF) stimulate clonal growth of nonhematopoietic tumor cells. *Blood*, 73: 80–3.

Carmo-Pereira, J., Costa, F.O., Henriques, E. *et al.* (1987). A comparison of two doses of Adriamycin in the primary chemotherapy of disseminated breast carcinoma. *Br. J. Cancer*, 56: 471–3.

Clark, G., Sledge, G.W., Osborne, C.K. & McGuire, W.L. (1987). Survival from first recurrence: relative importance of prognostic factors in 1015 breast cancer patients. *J. Clin. Oncol.* 5: 55–61.

Cohen, M., Rajendra, R. Ahuja, N., & Nguyen, D. (1990). Chemotherapy dose intensity and median survival in advanced breast cancer: no apparent relationship. *Proc Am. Soc. Clin. Oncol*, 9: 34.

Cote, R.J., Rosen, P.F., Lessor, M.N., Old, L.J. & Osbourne, M.P. (1991). Prediction of early relapse in patients with operable breast cancer by detection of occult bone marrow micrometastases. *J. Clin. Oncol.*, 9: 1749–56.

Crouse, D.A., Changnian, L., Kessinger, A., Ogren, F. & Sharp, J.G. (1990). Modulation of stem and progenitor cell number in the marrow, spleen and peripheral blood of tumor bearing mice. *J. Cell. Biochem.*, 14A: 326.

Dedhar, S., Gaboury, L., Galloway, P. & Eaves, C. (1988). Human granulocyte-macrophage colony-stimulating factor is a growth factor active on a variety of cell types of nonhemopoietic origin. *Proc. Natl. Acad. Sci. USA*, 85: 9253–7.

Demetri, G.D., Young, D.C., Merica, E. *et al.* (1991a). Clinical effects of interleukin-3 (IL-3) in patients with advanced sarcomas: a phase I/II trial. *Blood*, 78 (suppl. 1): 12 (abstract).

Demetri, G.D., Younger, J., McGuire, B.W. *et al.* (1991b). Recombinant methionyl granulocyte-CSF (G-CSF) allows an increase in the dose intensity of cyclophosphamide, doxorubicin, 5-fluorouracil (CAF) in patients with advanced breast cancer. *Proc. Am. Soc. Clin. Oncol*, 10: 70 (abstract 153).

Eder, J.P., Elias, A., Shed, T.C. *et al.* (1990). A phase I/II study of cyclophosphamide, thiotepa and carboplatin with autologous bone marrow transplantation in solid tumor patients. *J. Clin. Oncol*, 8: 1239–45.

Elias, A., Ayash, L., Anderson, K. *et al.* (1991a). GM-CSF mobilized peripheral blood progenitor cell support after high dose chemotherapy for breast cancer: effect of GM-CSF post reinfusion. *Blood*, 400a (abstract 1590).

Elias, A., Eder, J.P., Shea, T., Begg, C.B., Frei III, E. & Antman, K. (1990). High-dose ifosfamide with mesna uroprotection: a phase I study. *J. Clin. Oncol.*, 8: 170–8.

Elias, A., Mazanet, R., Wheeler, C. *et al.* (1991b). Peripheral blood progenitor cells: two protocols using GM-CSF potentiated progenitor cell collection. In *Autologous Bone Marrow Transplantation,* ed. K.A. Dicke & J. Armitage. *Proceedings of the Fifth International Symposium*, University of Nebraska, Omaha. pp. 875–80.

Ellis, G., Ferguson, M., Yamanaka, E., Livingston, R.B. & Gown, A.M. (1989). Monoclonal antibodies for detection of occult carcinoma cells in bone marrow of breast cancer patients. *Cancer*, 63: 2509–14.

Frei III, E., Antman, K., Teicher, B., Eder, P., Schnipper, L. (1989). Bone marrow autotransplantation for solid tumors-prospects. *J. Clin. Oncol*, 7: 515–26.

146 K.H. Antman

Frei III, E. & Canellos, G.P. (1980). Dose, a critical factor in cancer chemotherapy. *Am. J. Med.*, **69**: 585–94.

Gianni, A.M., Siena, S., Bregni, M. *et al.* (1989a). Granulocyte-macrophage colony stimulating factor to harvest circulating hematopoetic stem cells for autotransplant. *Lancet*, **ii**: 580–5.

Gianni, A.M., Siena, S., Bregni, M. *et al.* (1989b). Very rapid and comprise hematapoietic reconstitution following myeloablative treatments: the role of circulating stem cells harvested after high dose cyclophosphamide and GM-CSF. In *Autologous Bone Marrow Transplantation*, ed. K. Dicke, G. Spitzer, S. Jagganath & M. Evinger-Hodges. *Proceedings of the Fourth International Symposium*. The University of Texas, MD Anderson Press, Houston, pp. 723–32.

Gianni, A.M., Siena, S. *et al.* (1989c). Rapid and complete hematapoietic reconstitution following combined transplantation of autologous blood and bone marrow cells. A changing role for high dose chemoradiotherapy. *Hematol. Oncol.*, **7**: 139–48.

Goldman, J.M., Tr'ng, K., Park, D., Spiers, A., Lowenthal, R., Ruutu, T. (1978). Collection, cryopreservation and subsequent viability of haemopoietic stem cells intended for treatment of chronic granulocytic leukaemia in blast-cell transformation. *Br. J. Haematol.*, **40**: 185–95.

Gorin, N.C., Coiffier, B. & Pico, J. (1990). Granulocyte-macrophage colony stimulating factor shortens aplasia during autologous bone marrow transplantation in non-Hodgkin's lymphoma. A randomized placebo-controlled double blind study. *Blood*, **76** (suppl. 1): 542a.

Griffin, J.D., Spertini, O., Ernst, T.J., *et al.* (1990). Granulocyte-macrophage colony-stimulating factor and other cytokines regulate surface expression of the leukocyte adhesion molecule-1 on human neutrophils, monocytes, and their precursors. *J. Immunol.*, **145**: 576–84.

Henderson, I.C., Hayes, D.F. & Gelman, R. (1988). Dose-response in the treatment of breast cancer: a critical review. *J. Clin. Oncol*, **6**: 1501–15.

Herzig, G.P., Phillips, G.L., Herzig, R.H. *et al.* (1981). High dose nitrosourea and autologous bone marrow transplantation: a phase I trial. In *Nitrosoureas, Current Status and New Developments*, ed. C. Prestay Koaw & L.H. Bakes, pp. 337–41. Academic Press, New York.

Herzig, R.H., Fay, J.W., Herzig, G.P. *et al.* (1987). Phase I–II studies with high-dose thiotepa and autologous marrow transplantation in patients with refractory malignancies. In *Advances in Cancer Chemotherapy: High Dose Thiotepa and Autologous Marrow Transplantation*, ed. G.P. Herzig, Park Row Publishers, New York. pp. 17–33.

Hilkens, J., Buijs, F., Hilgers, J. *et al.* (1983). Monoclonal antibodies against human milk-fat globule membranes detecting differentiation antigens of the mammary gland and its tumors. *Int. J. Cancer.*, **34**: 197–206.

Hillner, B.E., Smith, T.J. & Desch, D.E. (1991). Estimating the cost-effectiveness of autologous bone marrow transplantation for metastatic breast cancer. *Proc. Am. Soc. Clin. Oncol.*, **10**: 46 (abstract 60).

Ho, J.Q.K., Juttner, C.A., To, L.B. *et al.* (1990). The threshold effect in peripheral blood stem cell autografting –differences between acute myeloid leukaemia and non 'stem cell disease'. *J. Cell Biochem.*, **14A**: 320.

Hryniuk, W.M. & Bush, H. (1984). The importance of dose intensity in chemotherapy of metastatic breast cancer. *J. Clin. Oncol.*, **2**: 1281–7.

Ingle, J.N., Tormey, D.C. & Tan, K.H. (1978). The bone marrow examination in breast cancer: diagnostic considerations and clinical usefulness. *Cancer*, **41**: 670–4.

Juttner, C.A., Haylock, D.N., Branford, A. *et al.* (1986). Haemopoietic reconstitution using circulating autologous stem cells collected in very early remission from acute non-lymphoblastic leukemia. *Exp. Hematol.*, **14**: 465 (abstract 312).

Kessinger, A., Armitage, A., Landmark, J. & Weisenberger, G. (1986). Reconstitution of human hematopoietic function with autologous cryopreserved circulating stem cells. *Exp. Hematol.*, **14**: 192–6.

Kessinger, A., O'Kane-Murphy, B., Jackson, J. *et al.* (1992). A comparison of different cryomedia and methods of freezing human hematopoietic stem cells from bone marrow and peripheral blood for storage. *Int. J. Cell Cloning*, **10** (suppl. 1): 88–91.

Kufe, D., Inghirami, G., Hayes, A.M., Wheeler, J. & Schlom, J. (1984). Differential reactivity of a novel monoclonal antibody (DF3) with human malignant versus benign breast tumors. *Hybridoma*, **3**: 223–32.

Link, H., Boogaerts, M., Carella, A. *et al.* (1990). Recombinant human granulocyte-macrophage colony stimulating factor after autologous bone marrow transplantation for acute lymphoblastic leukemia and non-Hodgkin's lymphoma: a randomized double blind multicenter trial in Europe. *Blood*, **76** (suppl. 1): 152a.

Lohrmann, H.P., Schreml, W., Lang, M., Betzler, M., Fliedner, T.M. & Heimpel, H. (1978). Changes of granulopoiesis during and after adjuvant chemotherapy of breast cancer. *Br. J. Haematol.*, **40**: 369–81.

Mann, S.L., Joshi, S.S., Weissenberger, D.D. *et al.* (1986). Detection of tumor cells in histologically normal bone marrow of autologous transplant patients using culture techniques. *Exp. Hematol.*, **14**: 541 (abstract 771).

Masaoka, T., Takaku, F., Kato, S. *et al.*, (1990). Recombinant human granulocyte colony stimulating factor for allogeneic bone marrow transplantation. *Proc Am. Assoc. Cancer Res.*, **31**: 173 (abstract 1028).

Mazanet, R., Elias, A., Hunt, M. *et al.* (1991). Peripheral blood progenitor cells (PBPC)s added to bone marrow (BM) for hemopoietic rescue following high dose chemotherapy for solid tumors reduces morbidity and length of hospitalization. *Proc. Am. Soc. Clin. Oncol.*, **10**: 324 (abstract 1140).

Michon, J., Bouffet, E., Bernard, J.L. *et al.* (1990). Administration of recombinant human GM-CSF (rHuGM-CSF) after autologous bone marrow transplantation (ABMT). A study of 21 stage IV neuroblastoma patients undergoing a double intensification regimen. *Proc. Am. Soc. Clin. Oncol.*, **9**: 184 (abstract 712).

Mick, R., Begg, C.B., Antman, K., Korzun, A.H. & Frei III, E. (1989). Diverse prognosis in metastatic breast cancer: who should be offered alternative initial therapies? *Breast Cancer Res. Treat.*, **13**: 33–38.

Nemunaitis, J., Rabinowe, S.N., Singer, J.W. *et al.* (1991). Recombinant granulocyte-macrophage colony-stimulating factor after autologous bone marrow transplantation for lymphoid malignancy: pooled results from three randomized double-blind, placebo controlled trials. *N. Engl. J. Med.*, **324**: 1773–8.

Norton, L. & Day, R. (1991). Potential innovations in scheduling of cancer chemotherapy. In *Important Advances in Oncology*, ed. V.T. De Vita Jr., S. Hellman & S.A. Rosenberg, pp. 57–72. J.B. Lippincott, Phildelphia.

Peters, W.P., Kurtzberg, I., Kirkpatrick, G. *et al.* (1989). GM-CSF primed peripheral blood progenitor cells (PBPC) coupled with autologous bone marrow transplantation (ABMT) will eliminate absolute leukopenia following high dose chemotherapy (HDC). *Blood*, **74**: 50 (abstract 178).

Philip, T., Michon, J., Gentet, J. *et al.* (1989). Use of GM-CSF in the LMCE double graft program for stage IV neuroblastoma: a blind study on 20 consecutive patients. *Proceedings of European Bone Marrow Transplantation.* Abstract 275.

Ravagnani, F., Siena, S., Beregni, M., Sciorelli, G., Gianni, A. & Pellegris, G. (1990). Large scale collection of circulating hematopoietic stem cells after high-dose cyclophosphamide cancer therapy and recombinant human GM-CSF. *Eur. J. Cancer*, **26**: 562–4.

Redding, W.H., Monaghan, P., Imrie, S.F. *et al.* (1983). Detection of micrometastases in patients with primary breast cancer. *Lancet*, **2**: 1271–4.

Richman, C.M., Weiner, R.S. & Yankee, R.A. (1976). Increase in circulating stem cells following chemotherapy in man. *Blood*, **47**: 1031–9.

Ruse-Riol, F., Legros, M., Bernard, D. *et al.* (1984). Variations in committed stem cells in the peripheral blood of cancer patients treated by sequential combination chemotherapy for breast cancer. *Cancer Res.*, **44**: 2219–24.

Sarpel, S.C., Axel, Z., Harrath, L. *et al.* (1979). The collection, preservation and function of peripheral blood hematopoietic cells in dogs. *Exp. Hematol.*, **7**: 113–20.

Schilder, R., LaCreta, F.P., Nash, S., Hudas, G.R., Ozals, R.F. & O'Dwyer, P.J. (1991). Phase 1 trial of thiotepa in combination with recombinant human GM-CSF. *Blood*, **78**: 7a.

Schilder, R.J., Nash, S., Tew, K.D., Panting, L., Comis, R.L. & O'Dwyer, P.J. (1990). Phase I trial of thiotepa (TT) in combination with the glutathione transferase (GST) inhibitor ethacrynic acid (EA). *Proc. Am. Assoc. Cancer Res.*, **31**: 177 (abstract 1051).

Sharp, J.G., Kessinger, A., Vaughan, W.P. *et al.* (1992). Detection and clinical significance of minimal tumor cell contamination of peripheral blood stem cell harvests. *Int. J. Cell Cloning*, **10** (suppl. 1): 92–4.

Shea, T., Mason, J., Storniolo, A. *et al.* (1990). Beneficial effect from sequential harvesting and reinfusing of peripheral blood stem cells in conjunction with rHu GM-CSF and high dose carboplatin. *Blood*, **26**: 165A.

Siena, S., Bregni, M., Brando, B., Ravagnani, F., Bonadonna, G. & Gianni, A. (1989). Circulation of CD34-positive hematopoietic stem cells in the peripheral blood of high-dose cyclophosphamide treated patients: enhancement by intravenous recombinant human GM-CSF. *Blood*, **74**: 1095–14.

Socinski, M.A., Cannistra, S.A., Ehas, A., Antman, K.H., Schnipper, L. & Griffin, J.D. (1988). Granulocyte-macrophage colony stimulating factor expands the circulating haemopoietic progenitor cell compartment in man. *Lancet*, **1**: 1194–8.

Spitzer, G., Buzdar, A., Auber, M. *et al.* (1987). High dose cyclophosphamide/VP-16/platinum intensification for metastatic breast cancer. *Breast Cancer Res. Treat.*, **10**: 89.

Tannock, I.F., Boyd, N.F., Deboer, G. *et al.* (1988). A randomized trial of two dose levels of cyclophosphamide, methotrexate, and fluorouracil chemotherapy for patients with metastatic breast cancer. *J. Clin. Oncol.*, **6**: 1377–87.

To, L.B., Haylock, D.N., Kimber, R. & Juttner, C.A. (1984). High levels of circulating hematopoietic stem cells in very early remission from acute non-lymphocytic leukaemia and their collection and cryopreservation. *Br. J. Haematol.*, **58**: 399–410.

To, L.B. & Juttner, C.A. (1987). Peripheral blood stem cell autografting: a new therapeutic option for AML? *Br. J. Haematol.*, **66**: 285–8.

Toki, H., Shimokawa, T., Okabe, K. & Ishimitsu, T. (1990). Recombinant human granulocyte colony-stimulating factor (rG-CSF) amplifies the number of peripheral blood stem cell (PBSC) of lymphoma patients on chemotherapy. *Proc Am. Soc. Clin. Oncol.*, **9**: 188 (abstract 728).

Vaughan, W., Mann, S., Garfrey, J. *et al.* (1990). Breast cancer detected in cell culture of histologically negative bone marrow predicts systemic relapse in patients with stage I, II, III, and locally recurrent disease. *Proc. Am. Assoc. Clin. Oncol.*, **9**: 9 (abstract 27).

Weiner, R., Richman, C. & Yankee, R. (1977). Semicontinuous flow centrifugation for the pheresis of immunocompetent cells and stem cells. *Blood*, **49**: 391–7.

Wolff, S., Herzig, R.H., Fay, J.W. *et al.* (1989). High dose thiotepa with ABMT for metastatic malignant melanoma: results of phase I and II studies of the North American BMT group. *J. Clin. Oncol.*, **7**: 245–9.

13

Blood stem cell transplants in myeloma

B. BARLOGIE, J.-P. FERMAND, P. HENON, J. REIFFERS AND S. JAGANNATH

Introduction

During the past decade, intensive chemotherapy has been investigated in multiple myeloma in order to achieve more marked tumor cytoreduction and, as a result, hopefully more durable disease control and possibly cure (McElwain & Powles, 1983; Barlogie et al., 1986, 1987, 1988, 1990; Harousseau et al., 1987, 1992; Selby et al., 1987; Gore et al., 1989; Jagannath et al., 1990; Anderson et al., 1991; Barlogie & Gahrton, 1991). The majority of studies employed autologous bone marrow and recent emphasis has been placed on blood stem cell transplants (for review, see Barlogie & Gahrton, 1991). The underlying rationale included: (1) lower frequency of myeloma cells in blood compared with bone marrow (an assumption still being debated) (Barlogie et al., 1989) and (2) the presence also of more mature hematopoietic progenitor cells, so that the duration of severe pancytopenia would be shortened. Blood stem cell procurement and engraftment have been further facilitated through the use of hematopoietic growth factors (Gianni et al. 1989). This chapter addresses the results of clinical trials in multiple myeloma with at least 20 patients in terms of blood stem cell procurement, posttransplant engraftment and anti-tumor effects.

Blood stem cell collection

Most studies in multiple myeloma have applied chemotherapy to increase the frequency of circulating hematopoietic stem cells (Henon et al., 1988, 1992; Fermand et al., 1989, 1992; Reiffers et al., 1989a, b; Ventura et al., 1990; Jagannath et al., 1991, 1992). Table 13.1 summarizes the use of single alkylating agent chemotherapy with cyclophosphamide or melphalan as well as combination chemotherapy with CHOP (cyclophosphamide, hydroxydaunorubicin, vincristine and prednisone). In Fermand's series (see Fermand *et al.*, 1992), blood stem cell collection could not be accomplished in 3 of 44 subjects with minimal or no prior therapy compared with 9 of 26 among cases with more than three courses of prior treatment. Blood stem cell collection after melphalan, targeting a more primitive hematopoietic stem cell, was associated, not surprisingly, with a lower success rate of 50% in procuring a sufficient quantity of blood stem cells (Henon *et al.*, 1992). In Jagannath's series of 75 patients, stem cell mobilization was judged by colony-forming unit granulocyte/macrophage (CFU-GM) and CD34 quantities in relationship to 10^5 mononuclear cells collected (Jagannath, 1991, 1992). 'Good' blood stem cell mobilization was accomplished overall in only about one-half of patients but in 85% of those who were not exposed to more than 12 months of prior therapy. Similarly, 85% of patients with rapid platelet recovery ($> 50 \times 10^9$/l) within 2 weeks after high dose cyclosphosphamide had 'good' stem cell mobilization as opposed to only 24% of those with slow platelet recovery. Granulocyte/macrophage colony-stimulating factor (GM-CSF) after high dose cyclosphosphamide facilitated blood stem cell mobilization both in the more extensively treated group of patients and in those with up to 12 months of prior therapy (Table 13.2). Similar quantities of nucleated cells (per kilogram body weight) could be procured with and without GM-CSF, the stem cell yield (by CFU-GM or CD34 expression) was consistently higher when GM-CSF was used (Table 13.3).

For successful blood stem cell collection prior treatment should be limited, especially with agents inflicting early stem cell damage such as melphalan. Melphalan treatment achieved a marked anti-tumor effect (7 of 20 patients with complete remission in Henon's series compared with 2 of 68 evaluated patients receiving high dose cyclosphosphamide in Jagannath's group), but it induced severe bone marrow aplasia of unpredictable duration and is therefore not recommended as a facilitator of blood stem cell mobilization and collection. Stem cell-sparing agents such as cyclophosphamide (Reiffers *et al.*, 1989b), etoposide and combinations such as CHOP or high dose cyclosphosphamide-VP16 (Glenn *et al.*, 1991), in contrast are compatible with adequate blood stem cell collection and low treatment-related mortality in the 2–5% range as opposed to 15% in the case of melphalan. Administration of hematopoietic growth factors, such as GM-CSF or granulocyte colony-stimulating factor (G-CSF), further enhance blood stem cell mobilization (Tables 13.2 and 13.3).

When there was doubt about hematopoietic stem cell reserve in a given patient with prior chemotherapy, high dose cyclosphosphamide proved to

Table 13.1. *Blood-stem cell collection for myeloma*

| Author | Regimen | Number of patients | | | Successful BSC collection[a] |
		Total	Limited prior therapy	Myeloma stage III	
Reiffers	HD CY 7 g/m^2	26	22	23	17
Henon	MEL 100–140 mg/m^2	20	6	20	10
Fermand	CHOP CY × 4 g/m^2, ADR 100 mg/m^2	73	46 29	73	58
Jagannath	HD CY 6 g/m^2 ± GM-CSF	75	≤12 months 31 resistant to MP and VAD	NA in previously treated patients	40

ADR, Adriamycin® (doxorubicin hydrochloride); BSC, blood stem cell; CHOP, cyclophosphamide, hydroxydaunorubicin, vincristine and prednisone; HD CY, high dose cyclophosphamide; MEL, melphalan; NA, not applicable; MP, melphalan and prednisolone; VAD, vincristine, adriamycin and dexamethasone; TE, too early; F/U, follow-up; VP16, etoposide.
[a] > 2 × 10^4 CFU-GM/kg body weight in the series by Reiffers, Henon and Fermand; > 50 CFU-GM per 10^5, mononuclear cells collected in Jagannath's series, although 72 of 75 patients had PBSC collection.

Table 13.2. *Factors affecting blood stem cell collection in Jagannath's series*

Months of prior therapy	GM-CSF	Number	Patients with 'good' BSC[a] (%)
> 12	−	25	28
> 12	+	20	50
≤ 12	−	11	73
≤ 12	+	16	94

[a] > 50 CFU-GM per 10^5 mononuclear cells (Jagannath *et al.*, 1992).
BSC, blood stem cell; CFU-GM, colony-forming unit-granulocyte/macrophage; GM-CSF, granulocyte/macrophage colony-stimulating factor.

be a valuable *in vivo* stress test. Rapid platelet recovery to $50 \times 10^9/l$ within 2 weeks from high dose cyclosphosphamide was indicative of adequate stem cell mobilization, which in turn assured prompt engraftment after high dose therapy (see below). Patients with poor stem cell yield could be excluded from marrow-ablative transplant regimens.

There is only limited and unpublished experience in multiple myeloma with blood stem cell mobilization using hematopoietic growth factors alone without chemotherapy priming. Such approaches, especially with IL-3 and GM-CSF, are anticipated to further reduce the risk of infection and bleeding.

Transplant regimens and engraftment

Preparative regimens varied among the different trials reviewed here, including melphalan (140 mg/m²) plus total body irradiation (1200 cGy) in six fractions (Reiffers *et al.*, 1989a); melphalan (280 mg/m²) plus total body irradiation (1000 cGy) in six fractions (Henon *et al.*, 1988, 1992); melphalan (140 mg/m²) plus total body irradiation (1200 cGy) and added carmustine (120 mg/m²), etoposide (750 mg/m²) with or without cyclophosphamide (2400 mg/m²) (Barlogie *et al.*, 1986, 1987, 1988, 1989, 1990; Harousseau *et al.*, 1987, 1992; Selby *et al.*, 1987; Henon *et al.*, 1988; Fermand *et al.*, 1989, 1992; Gianni *et al.*, 1989; Gore *et al.*, 1989; Reiffers *et al.*, 1989a; Jagannath *et al.*, 1990; Anderson *et al.*, 1991; Barlogie & Gahrton, 1991); and melphalan (200 mg/m²) or melphalan (140 mg/m²) and total body irradiation (850 cGy) (Jagannath *et al.*, 1991, 1992) (Table 13.4). The proportion of patients receiving transplants varied from 100%

Table 13.3. *High dose cyclophosphamide with or without GM-CSF and blood stem cell collection*

Author	High dose cyclophosphamide (g/m^2)	GM-CSF	Number	Cell yield × 10^8/kg bw (range)	CFU-GM × 10^4/kg bw (mean)	p value
Reiffers	7	+	8	7 (1.2–24.6)	15.6 (0.7–286)	0.03
		–	8	6.2 (2.7–13.1)	1.6 (0.1–33.9)	
Jagannath	6	+	36	7.3 (3.6–13.1)	44 (2.1–129)	<0.001
		–	36	6.8 (2.5–17.2)	17 (1.1–50.3)	

bw = body weight; for other abbreviations see Table 13.2.

Table 13.4. *Attrition of patients from blood stem cell collection to transplant*

Author	Transplant regimen MEL (mg/m²)	TBI (cGy)	Other	Enrolled for BSC mobilization	trans-planted	ABMT added	TE	Deaths Prior to Tx[a]	During Tx	Median days to Granulocytes >500 ×10⁶/l	Platelets >50 ×10⁹/l
Reiffers	140	1200	HD CY in 3 patients	26	26	7	0	0	0	13	28
Henon	280	1000	—	20	10	1	0	3	1	11	22
Fermand	140	1200	HD CY 2.4 g/m² CCNU 120 mg/m² VP16 750 mg/m²	73	43	?	6	5	3	15	29
Jagannath	140 200	— —	Busulfan 16 mg/kg	75	7 57	NA	NA	NA	NA	NA	NA
	140	850	± GM-CSF		57 3	57	9	3	0	15	19

BSC, blood stem cell; ABMT, autologous bone marrow transplant; GM-CSF, granulocyte/macrophage colony-stimulating factor; HD CY, high dose cyclophosphamide; CCNU, lomustine; VP16, etoposide; MEL, melphalan; NA, not available; TE, too early; TBI, total body irradiation; Tx = treatment.

[a]Includes deaths during BSC collection, from disease progression while awaiting transplantation or from other causes.

B. Barlogie et al.

Table 13.5. *Posttransplant engraftment in Jagannath's series*

GM-CSF post HD-CY	Months from first treatment	Number	Granulocytes $> 500 \times 10^6/l$	Platelets $> 50 \times 10^9/l$
−	>12	18	20	32
−	≤12	11	19	21
+	>12	15	15	17
+	≤12	16	14	15

For abbreviations see Table 13.4.

in Reiffers' series to a low of 50% in Henon's study. Two-thirds of Fermand's and 80% of Jagannath's initial patients proceeded to transplantation with additional patients still awaiting transplants. Only the latter series employed, by design, autologous bone marrow in addition to blood stem cells in the majority of patients; GM-CSF was used for blood stem cell mobilization in 36 patients and posttransplant in 38 patients; all stem cells were obtained prior to the first transplant.

Hematologic recovery of the transplanted patients was relatively uniform for granulocyte levels, reaching $500 \times 10^6/l$, which was accomplished within 11 to 15 days (Table 13.4). Even patients with limited prior therapy receiving GM-CSF in Jagannath's series required 15 days to reach such granulocyte levels. Safe platelet levels of at least $50 \times 10^9/l$ were not reached until 4 weeks after transplantation except in the Jagannath and Henon series (medians of 19 and 22 days, respectively). In the former study, platelet and granulocyte recovery proceeded equally fast within 2 weeks in the subgroup of patients with limited prior treatment exposure who also received GM-CSF for blood stem cell mobilization (Table 13.5). This experience was shared by Reiffers *et al.* (1989a, b), who noted further acceleration of engraftment when GM-CSF was used in conjunction with HD-CTX for blood stem cell collection. Fifty of 60 transplanted patients achieved complete hematologic recovery (as defined by granulocytes $> 1.5 \times 10^9/l$, platelets $> 100 \times 10^9/l$ and hemoglobin > 10 g/dl) within 1 month.

Anti-tumor effect

The anti-tumor activity of blood stem cell mobilization regimens was generally limited, except when melphalan was used at a dose of 100–140 mg/m² (35% complete remission); high dose cyclosphosphamide at 6 g/m² effected a 38% response rate (cytoreduction by at least 75%) among 37 evaluated patients with responsive multiple myeloma, compared with only 16% in 31 subjects with refractory disease ($p = 0.05$) (Jagannath *et al.*, 1991, 1992).

Reiffers (1989a) observed 23 responses among 26 patients treated with transplants including 13 complete remissions (Table 13.6). With a median follow-up of 18 months (range 4–41 months), 18 patients remain relapse-free, while 8 have relapsed after 3–34 months (median 22 months). Overall median survival is projected to be 36 months, with 65% of patients still alive. Henon *et al.* (1992) noted 9 complete remissions and 1 partial remission (in the 1 patient who also received autologous marrow transplant); 1 treatment-related death occurred at 45 days; 2 patients died from unrelated causes; and 2 patients relapsed 12 and 24 months posttransplant. Six patients remain alive at 4, 5, 8, 13, 38 and 48 months, five of whom are in unmaintained complete remission 4–38 months after transplant (Henon *et al.*, 1992). Of 20 patients initially enrolled, six (30%) were alive at the last follow-up. The median survival of 22 months in the 10 transplanted patients significantly exceeded the 14 months of the 7 nontransplanted subjects ($p = 0.02$).

In Fermand's series of 73 patients (Fermand *et al.*, 1989, 1992), 3 died during high dose CHOP-induced aplasia; 58 of the remaining 70 patients had adequate blood stem cells, of whom 6 are still awaiting transplants at the time of their relapse (Table 13.6). Two patients died from progressive multiple myeloma before transplant and 7 were treated with busulfan and melphalan. Of the remaining 43 patients treated with total body irradiation-containing preparative regimens, 3 died from marrow aplasia and 1 from infection 5 months posttransplant. All 39 evaluated patients responded. After a median follow-up of 35 months posttransplant (range 9–70 months), 10 patients relapsed of whom 4 died at 18, 19, 20 and 44 months. Thus, of 43 patients receiving total body irradiation, there have been 8 deaths and 6 relapses for 14 events. The 4-year survival and event-free survival estimates are 73% and 50%, respectively. Considering all 73 patients, the median survival is projected to be 5 years, with 66% of patients still alive.

In Jagannath's series of 75 patients receiving high dose cyclosphosphamide, 72 underwent blood stem cell collection, of whom 2 died prior to transplant and 1 received an allogeneic bone marrow transplant (Jagannath *et al.*, 1991, 1992). Nine are still awaiting autologous transplants. After transplant, 45 of 60 patients were in remission ($\geqslant 75\%$ regression) and 12 in complete

Table 13.6. *Clinical outcome after blood stem cell-supported intensive therapy*

Author	Number of patients		Deaths pre- and peri-treatment	Response[a]	Complete remission[b]	Median months of F/U	Current status of all patients
	Total	Treatment					
Reiffers	26	26	0	23	13	18	Median survival, 36 months 65% alive
Henon	20	10	4[c]	10	9	?	30% alive
Fermand	73	50	8	39/39[d]	?	35	Median survival, 60 months 66% alive
Jagannath	75	60	3	45[e]	12[e]	10	83% alive
		32[f]	0	29[g]	12[g]	12	91% alive

[a]Variable, ≥ 50 or $\geq 75\%$ cytoreduction.
[b]Complete remission (CR), usually immunofixation negative and normal bone marrow.
[c]2 deaths from unrelated events in CR 10 and 18 months post transplant.
[d]Responses per number of evaluable patients.
[e]Response after one transplant.
[f]Second transplant.
[g]Response after two transplants (second transplant: melphalan (200 mg/m^2) on day 26; melphalan and total body irradiation in five fractions; cyclophosphamide, etoposide (VP-16), total body irradiation in one fraction).

remission. The study design called for a second transplant, which has so far been performed in 32 patients 3–12 months later (median 4 months; 84% within 6 months). As a result, the complete remission rate increased from 25% after the first to 38% after the second transplant. With a median follow-up of 10 months, 83% remain alive with event-free and overall survival projections at 12 months of 86% and 88%, respectively.

Discussion and summary

Autologous blood stem cells are increasingly being employed to support high dose and even marrow-ablative therapy for multiple myeloma. Compared with autologous bone marrow, more patients can potentially benefit from blood stem cells if one considers that approximately 30–40% of newly diagnosed patients do not respond to induction therapy and hence do not achieve a bone marrow remission. Fewer patients probably have persistent marrow plasmacytosis in excess of 30%, and several autologous marrow transplant trials have not reported an adverse influence of autografts containing up to 30% tumor cells. Compared with bone marrow collection, blood stem cell collection is more time-consuming but does not require general anesthesia. Blood stem cells represent the hematopoietic stem cell source of choice in case of extensive prior pelvic irradiation or persistent marrow plasmacytosis of more than 30%.

Procurement of blood stem cells can be done in several ways, i.e. under steady state conditions (Kessinger & Armitage, 1991), using chemotherapy priming with or without growth factor support and with growth factor support alone without preceding chemotherapy. As with bone marrow autografts, CFU-GM serve as a first approximation in judging the quality of blood stem cells. There was no disparity between the incidence of successful hematopoietic stem cell procurement from bone marrow and blood. Patients with 'good' mobilization (>50 CFU-GM/10^5 mononuclear cells) had significantly higher bone marrow CFU-GM (3×10^4/kg body weight) compared with those with 'poor' blood stem cell collection (1.2×10^4/kg body weight) ($p < 0.0001$).

Impairment of blood stem cell (and also bone marrow stem cell) collection results from prolonged prior therapy especially with alkylating agents targeting immature stem cells. Among subjects with limited prior treatment (up to 12 months in Jagannath's series), adequate quantities and qualities of stem cells could be collected in 73–94%, depending on whether GM-CSF was employed. Melphalan is not recommended for blood stem cell mobilization as only 50% of patients were candidates for subsequent blood stem cell collection (Henon *et al.*, 1992). These data are reminiscent of results reported by Harousseau's group using melphalan as a highly effective initial treatment with the intent of *in vivo* purging of autologous bone marrow (Harousseau *et al.*, 1987, 1992). Additional disadvantages of the melphalan approach include a considerable mortality rate of about 15% as opposed to less than 5% with other priming regimens and the preclusion of any hematopoietic stem cell-supported therapy in about one-half of the patients. GM-CSF and possibly other growth factors facilitate blood stem cell collection after high dose cyclosphosphamide or similar stem cell-sparing regimens, so that the number of apheresis procedures can be reduced to approximately two to three runs.

Granulocyte recovery to at least $500 \times 10^6/l$ after transplantation proceeded within 2 weeks when sufficient stem cell quantities were employed. Platelet recovery to $50 \times 10^9/l$ was delayed to about 4 weeks but proceeded within 3 weeks when GM-CSF was used for blood stem cell mobilization. In fact, recovery to normal blood counts was noted within 1 month in 50 of 60 patients receiving both marrow and blood stem cells. Similar information is not available for blood stem cell-supported therapies, although studies in other malignancies seem to indicate that blood affords complete engraftment similar to bone marrow (Kessinger & Armitage, 1991).

Any anti-tumor effect depends on the conditioning regimen employed, the stage of myeloma at presentation, presence of resistance to prior standard therapy, and possibly on the source of hematopoietic stem cells and the use of potentially growth-stimulating growth factors (Jagannath & Barlogie, 1992). Single transplants appear most effective when total body irradiation is part of the regimen, as evidenced by a high complete remission rate (although this definition is not uniform among the reviewed studies). The majority of patients in the series of Reiffers, Henon and Fermand had recently diagnosed multiple myeloma, although of advanced state, so that complete remission rates in the 50% range are not surprising and were reminiscent of results achieved with autologous marrow transplants in support of total body irradiation-containing regimens for similar patients (Attal *et al.*, 1992; Jagannath *et al.*, 1992). By contrast, Jagannath's study included 31 patients with multiple myeloma refractory to both standard alkylating agents and VAD, explaining the low incidence of complete remission of only 8%. In the subset of 27 patients treated within 6 months from diagnosis and receiving, by design, two transplants, 11 achieved true complete remission and had prompt and complete hematopoietic reconstitution. The toxicity of each transplant was reduced by avoiding the use of total body irradiation and by the combined use of marrow and blood stem cells with GM-CSF.

Fermand's series has the longest follow-up, with a median of 35 months. Survival rates of 60% at 2 years and 50% at 5 years are similar to results reported with melphalan and total body irradiation with autologous bone marrow grafts in similar patients (Jagannath *et al.*, 1990; Attal *et al.*, 1992; Jagannath & Barlogie, 1992). Using such chemoradiotherapy as remission consolidation or even for primary refractory multiple myeloma, early mortality was under 5% and 4-year projections of relapse-free and overall survival were at 45% and 65%, respectively, with a minimum follow-up of 26 months.

Experience from a single investigator team, originally employing autologous bone marrow transplants alone without hematopoietic growth factors to support melphalan and total body irradiation and who now use bone marrow and blood stem cells with GM-CSF in support of double transplants suggests that the latter approach affords granulocyte recovery ($> 500 \times 10^6$/l) within 2 weeks and platelet recovery ($> 50 \times 10^9$/l) in 3 weeks. This is 1–2 weeks earlier than with bone marrow alone (Jagannath *et al.*, 1990, 1991, 1992). With blood stem cells, there was no transplant-related mortality although one death occurred in conjunction with blood stem cell procurement and two further patients died while awaiting transplants (see Table 13.5).

Compared with bone marrow autografts (Jagannath *et al.*, 1990; Barlogie & Gahrton, 1991) and blood stem cells collected under steady state conditions (Lobo *et al.*, 1991), chemotherapy-primed blood stem cell collection shortened severe neutropenia by at least 1 week and virtually eliminated peritransplant mortality. The important issue of less tumor cell reseeding from blood stem cell compared with bone marrow has not yet been addressed. Extensive laboratory studies, however, leave no doubt about circulating tumor cells, apparently at a relatively early stage of maturation. Gene transfer studies should permit elucidation of the relative contributions to relapse from bone marrow and blood stem cell autografts (Buschle *et al.*, 1991).

Acknowledgements

The authors gratefully acknowledge the excellent technical assistance of Dwayne Bracy and Paula Owen and the dedicated secretarial assistance of Angie Woodliff.

References

Anderson, K., Barut, B., Ritz, J. *et al.* (1991). Monoclonal antibody purged autologous bone marrow transplantation for multiple myeloma. *Blood*, **77**: 712–20.

Attal, M., Huguet, F., Schlaifer, D. *et al.* (1992). Intensive combined therapy for previously untreated aggressive myeloma. *Blood*, **79**: 1130–6.

Barlogie, B. & Gahrton, G. (1991). Bone marrow transplantation in multiple myeloma – a review. *Bone Marrow Transplant*, **7**: 71–9.

Barlogie, B., Alexandian, R., Dicke, K. *et al.* (1987). High dose chemoradiotherapy and autologous bone marrow transplantation for resistant multiple myeloma. *Blood*, **70**: 869–72.

Barlogie, B., Alexanian, R., Smallwood, L. *et al.* (1988). Prognostic factors with high dose melphalan for refractory multiple myeloma. *Blood*, **72**: 2015–19.

Barlogie, B., Epstein, J., Selvanayagam, P. & Alexanian, R. (1989). Plasma cell myeloma: new biological insights and advances in therapy. *Blood*, **73**, 865–79.

Barlogie, B., Hall, R., Zander, A. *et al.* (1986). High dose melphalan with autologous bone marrow transplantation for multiple myeloma. *Blood*, **67**: 1298–301.

Barlogie, B., Jagannath, S., Dixon, D. *et al.* (1990). High dose melphalan and GM-CSF for refractory multiple myeloma. *Blood*, **76**: 677–80.

Buschle, M., Campana, D., Hoffbrand, A.V. & Brenner, M.K. (1991). Transfection of human bone marrow B cell progenitors. *Blood*, **78** (suppl.): 311a.

Fermand, J.P., Levy, Y., Gerota, J. *et al.* (1989). Treatment of aggressive multiple myeloma by high-dose chemotherapy and total body irradiation followed by blood stem cell autologous graft. *Blood*, **73**: 20–3.

Fermand, J.P., Chevret, S., Levy, Y. *et al.* (1992). The role of autologous blood stem cells in support of high dose therapy for multiple myeloma. In *Hematology/Oncology Clinics of North America*, ed. B. Barlogie, pp. 451–62. W.B. Saunders, Philadelphia, PA.

Gianni, A.M., Siena, S., Bregni, M. *et al.* (1989). Granulocyte-macrophage colony-stimulating factor to harvest circulating haemopoietic stem cells for autotransplantation. *Lancet*, **ii**: 580–4.

Glenn, L.D., Jagannath, S., Vesole, D. & Barlogie, B. (1991). Mobilization of peripheral blood stem cells (PBSC-M) and response to high-dose cyclophosphamide (CY) and etoposide (VP-16). *Blood*, **78** (suppl.) 222a.

Gore, M.E., Selby, P.J., Viner, C. *et al.* (1989). Intensive treatment of multiple myeloma and criteria for complete remission. *Lancet*, **ii**: 879–85.

Harousseau, J.L., Milpied, N., Garand, R. & Bourhis, J.H. (1987). High dose melphalan and autologous bone marrow transplantation in high risk myeloma. *Br. J. Haematol.*, **67**: 493.

Harousseau, J.L., Milpied, N., Laporte, J.P. *et al.* (1992). Double intensive therapy in high risk multiple myeloma. *Blood*, **79**: 2827–33.

Henon, Ph., Beck, G., Debecker, A., Eisenmann, J.C., Lepers, M. & Kandel, G. (1988). Autograft using peripheral blood stem cells collected after high dose melphalan in high risk myeloma. *Br. J. Haematol.*, **71**: 253–4.

Henon, Ph., Eisenmann, J.C., Beck-Wirth, G. & Liang, H. (1992). A two-phase intensive therapeutic approach in high risk myeloma. Follow up. In *Proceedings of the Second International Symposium on Peripheral Blood Stem Cell Autografts*, ed. Ph. Henon & C. Juttner. *Int. J. Cell Cloning*, **10**: 142–4.

Jagannath, S. & Barlogie, B. (1992). Autologous bone marrow transplantation in multiple myeloma. In *Hematology/Oncology Clinics of North America*, ed. B. Barlogie, pp. 437–50. W.B. Saunders, Philadelphia, PA.

Jagannath, S., Vesole, D., Glenn, L. & Barlogie, B. (1991). High dose cyclophosphamide (HDCTX) for blood stem cell mobilization (BSCM) in patients with multiple myeloma. *Blood*, **78** (suppl.): 125a.

Jagannath, S., Vesole, D. & Barlogie, B. (1992). High dose therapy, autologous stem cells and hemopoietic growth factors for the management of multiple myeloma. In *High-Dose Cancer Therapy*, ed. J. Armitage, K. Antman, pp. 638–50. Williams and Wilkins, Baltimore, MD.

Jagannath, S., Barlogie, B., Dicke, K.A. *et al.* (1990). Autologous bone marrow transplantation in multiple myeloma: identification of prognostic factors. *Blood*, **76**: 1860–6.

Kessinger, A. & Armitage, J.O. (1991). The evolving role of autologous peripheral blood stem cell transplantation following high dose therapy for malignancies. *Blood*, **77**: 211–13.

Lobo, F., Kessinger, A., Landmark, J.D. *et al.* (1991). Addition of peripheral blood stem cells collected without mobilization techniques to transplanted autologous bone marrow did not hasten marrow recovery following myeloablative therapy. *Bone Marrow Transplant.*, **8**: 389–92.

McElwain, T.J. & Powles, R.L. (1983). High-dose intravenous melphalan for plasma-cell leukemia and myeloma. *Lancet*, **i**: 822–3.

Reiffers, J., Marit, G. & Bostron, J.M. (1989a). Autologous blood stem cell transplantation in high-risk multiple myeloma. *Br. J. Haematol.*, **72**: 296–7.

Reiffers, J., Marit, G. & Bostron, J.M. (1989b). Peripheral blood stem-cell transplantation in intensive treatment of multiple myeloma. *Lancet*, **ii**: 1336.

Selby, P., McElwain, T.J., Nandi, A.C. *et al.* (1987). Multiple myeloma treated with high dose intravenous melphalan. *Br. J. Haematol.*, **66**: 55–62.

Ventura, G.J., Barlogie, B., Hester, J.P. *et al.* (1990). High dose cyclophosphamide, BCNU and VP-16 with autologous blood stem cell support for refractory multiple myeloma. *Bone Marrow Transplant.*, **V**: 265–8.

Part III

Summary

14

Blood stem cell transplants: current state; future directions

C.A. JUTTNER, P. HENON AND R.P. GALE

High dose therapy

Current interest in blood stem cell transplants must be considered in the context of the efficacy of high dose therapy. Reviews by Hryniuk and colleagues suggest that intensity of conventional dose chemotherapy, i.e. delivered dose and time over which it is given, correlates with response rate in several cancers including breast, small cell lung, and ovarian cancer, Hodgkin's disease and nonHodgkin's lymphoma (Hryniuk, 1988). It is uncertain whether these increased response rates translate to more cures.

Less is known about higher dose therapy. Relapse is clearly further decreased in some patients receiving high dose therapy and allogeneic bone marrow transplants. Examples include acute and chronic myelogenous leukemia and acute lymphoblastic leukemia. In chronic myelogenous leukemia, but less certainly acute myelogenous leukemia and acute lymphoblastic leukemia, these decreased relapse risks translate to increased leukemia-free survival. It is uncertain, however, whether decreased relapse results from high dose therapy or immune-mediated anti-cancer effects collectively termed graft-versus-leukemia. Studies from the International Bone Marrow Transplant Registry comparing twin transplants, allogeneic conventional and T cell-depleted transplants without graft-versus-host disease suggest several immune-mediated anti-leukemia effects (Horowitz et al., 1990). Recent studies of donor blood cell infusions in patients with chronic myelogenous leukemia who relapse after high dose therapy and an allogeneic transplant support this notion (Kolb et al., 1990). The contribution of high dose therapy and autotransplants to decrease relapse and increase survival is even more unclear. While some studies report cures in advanced Hodgkin's disease and nonHodgkin's lymphoma, it is uncertain whether these results differ from chemotherapy alone.

The most convincing data supporting a benefit of high dose therapy and autotransplants comes from studies in advanced breast cancer (see Chapter 12 for a review).

Early studies in advanced nonHodgkin's lymphoma showed long-term benefit only in patients whose disease was responsive to conventional dose chemotherapy pretransplant. This may not be so in Hodgkin's disease, where there is some evidence of long-term benefit even in persons with resistant disease (Jagannath *et al.*, 1986). One study prospectively randomized patients with intermediate grade nonHodgkin's lymphoma that was still responsive to chemotherapy to conventional chemotherapy and total lymphoid irradiation or to high dose therapy and an autotransplant. No benefit is as yet reported for high dose therapy (Bron *et al.*, 1991). Another small unrandomized study of early high dose therapy and autotransplants in patients with intermediate grade lymphoma and poor prognostic features suggests a benefit for high dose therapy (Gulati *et al.*, 1988). Preliminary data from a similar study also suggest a benefit for intensive treatment (Gianni *et al.*, 1991).

What about blood stem cell transplants in the context of these data? If there are advantages for blood stem cells (see below), their possible role is to allow autotransplants in patients who may be older or sicker, or who have bone marrow metastasis, or who have received prior bone marrow irradiation.

Potential advantages of blood stem cells

Initial interest in blood stem cells centered on a postulated lower likelihood of contamination with cancer cells. Sharp and Kessinger (see Chapter 7) discuss this concept and the rather limited data currently available to test this notion. Clonogenicity (ability of tumour cells to grow *in vitro*) from bone marrow samples seems associated with a poor prognosis in breast cancer but not in Hodgkin's disease. Sharp and Kessinger provide a useful definition of minimal residual disease

minimal residual disease exists when the tumor cells remaining in the patient after therapy or present in hematopoietic stem cell harvests, not detectable by either standard clinical or histopathologic techniques, respectively may become a cause of relapse in the patient.

Implicit is the important issue of origin of relapse. Presently it is impossible to determine whether relapse after an autotransplant occurs because high dose therapy fails to eradicate all residual clonogenic cancer cells in the patient, because clonogenic tumour stem cells are reinfused with the graft, or both. It is not known whether there is less cancer in blood stem cell transplants, although Sharp and Kessinger present some data suggesting less tumor contamination in blood stem cell grafts.

Initial clinical studies of transplants showed consistent rapid hematopoietic reconstitution (Juttner *et al.*, 1985; Korbling *et al.*, 1986; Reiffers *et al.*, 1986). This was unexpected but probably predictable, given the increased numbers of late stem cells in the blood during rapid recovery from myelosuppressive chemotherapy. Initial reports of autotransplants of blood stem cells collected without prior chemotherapy or growth factors showed no acceleration of hematopoietic recovery compared with bone marrow autotransplants (Kessinger *et al.*, 1989). Preliminary data suggest that rapid hematopoietic recovery is predictable, resulting in fewer days with fever, fewer transfusions and briefer hospitalization (Elias *et al.*, 1992; To *et al.*, 1992). These all decrease cost, even when the expense of blood stem cell collection and cryopreservation procedures is considered. Some preliminary data suggest that immune reconstitution may also be accelerated by blood stem cell autotransplants (To *et al.*, 1987; Henon *et al.*, 1992). This might be important if immune anti-tumor effects operate after autotransplants.

Tumor contamination

Sharp and Kessinger (see Chapter 7) review current data concerning comparative malignant contamination of bone marrow and blood stem cell autografts. Important concepts are defined.

These authors review techniques to assess tumor contamination and discuss the concept of clonogenicity. They argue that phenotypic assessment of residual cancer cells fails to distinguish between tumor cells capable or not capable of causing relapse. Most phenotypic features are also markers of normal differentiation and it is impossible to be certain whether a specific marker or combination thereof precisely identifies a cancer cell capable of causing relapse. Combined studies of *ex vivo* growth and phenotype probably add sensitivity and specificity but remain imperfect.

Assessment of the genotype of residual cancer cells may hold more promise for assessing the importance of tumor contamination of the graft. The semiquantitative polymerase chain reaction has been successfully applied to BCR/ABL rearrangement in chronic myelogenous leukemia and the BCL2/IGH rearrangement in follicular lymphoma. Polymerase chain reaction technology, however, is often too sensitive and its use may be associated with frequent 'false positives'. Again, a distinction between cells capable of causing relapse or not is impossible with this technique. One study of autotransplants in low grade nonHodgkin's lymphoma suggests that detection of residual tumor cells in the graft using the polymerase chain reaction correlates with relapse (Gribben *et al.*, 1991). Most relapses, however, occurred in sites of prior disease. One explanation is that a positive polymerase chain reaction test is an overall prognostic factor independent of whether residual tumor cells in the graft cause relapse. Alternatively, infused tumor stem cells may 'home' in to sites of prior disease. It is more likely, however, that these sites contain residual cancer cells even after high dose therapy and that this is the cause of relapse. The patients reported were selected on the basis of responsiveness to chemotherapy. Low grade lymphomas are characteristically associated with a constant risk of relapse over many years. Critical analysis of this study is not presently possible because of these confounding issues.

Fluorescent *in situ* hybridization (FISH) of interphase cells is another technique used to assess cancer genotype. Studies of this are beginning in autotransplants for acute myeloid leukemia. These studies, however, are not able to distinguish relapse from residual leukemia in the patient and relapse from infused leukemia cells. Another approach is to use unique retroviral integration sites to 'mark' cancer cells. This may allow later determination of whether relapse results from the graft or from residual tumor in the patient (Brenner *et al.*, 1992). If only some infused cancer cells are clonogenic it will be important to establish ways of ensuring that all infused cells are 'marked'. This is not currently possible.

Despite these limitations some conclusions can be drawn from the initial clinical studies of blood stem cells autotransplants. Interestingly there may be increased disease-free survival in one study comparing blood stem cells with bone marrow transplants in patients with nonHodgkin's lymphoma without bone marrow involvement. Similar data have also been reported in women with breast cancer (see Chapter 7).

Are mobilized blood stem cells better?

The choice between unmobilized versus mobilized blood stem cells is in part determined by the study design. If the primary reason for using blood stem cells is to reduce tumor contamination of the graft in transplant patients with bone marrow metastasis, then stable-phase blood stem cell collection makes sense. If, however, the main reason for using blood stem cells is to expedite hematopoietic reconstitution posttransplant, then mobilized blood stem cells are probably better. Collecting blood stem cells after chemotherapy may achieve both objectives. In acute myeloid leukemia some data suggest that leukemia cells proliferate less rapidly than their normal counterparts and that early remission or postconsolidation blood stem cell collections may have lower likelihood of tumor contamination (To *et al.*, 1984). Alternatively, there may be a disadvantage to the approach as leukemia cells may be mobilized. Mobilization using hematopoietic growth factors may also increase tumor contamination with leukemia cells. G-CSF (granulocyte colony-stimulating factor) and GM-CSF (granulocyte/macrophage colony-stimulating factor) stimulate acute and chronic myeloid leukemia cells. Other data suggest that other cancers are stimulated by these factors. For example, GM-CSF and IL-6 (interleukin-6) stimulate *in vitro* growth of myeloma cells. Economic considerations are likely to lead to the increased use of mobilized blood stem cells alone or combined with bone marrow.

How should blood stem cells be mobilized?

Many studies have demonstrated that different chemotherapy regimens increase numbers of progenitor cells, like CFU-GM (colony-forming unit (granulocyte/macrophage)), in the blood during recovery from myelosuppression. Some drugs such as cyclophosphamide, cytarabine, daunorubicin and etoposide, regularly cause this effect. Others, such as melphalan, damage hematopoietic stem cells, rarely increase CFU-GM and are probably undesirable mobilizing agents. Use of chemotherapy to mobilize blood stem cells may be associated with additional anti-tumor effects. Chemotherapy, however, can result in substantial morbidity and even mortality (To *et al.*, 1990a). This factor should be included in the assessment of treatment schemes and cost.

Recent data indicate that G-CSF and, to a lesser extent GM-CSF, mobilize blood stem cells (Sheridan *et al.*, 1992; Socinski *et al.*, 1988). G-CSF mobilized blood stem cells are capable of early, intermediate and (in the mouse) long-term hematopoietic reconstitution. Most studies in humans using GM-CSF blood stem cells have also used bone marrow cells. Consequently, assessment of long-term reconstitution is not possible. Short-term reconstitution is generally satisfactory (Elias *et al.*, 1992). Combinations of cytokines given sequentially or simultaneously are being studied. Preliminary data in humans focus on IL-3 and GM-CSF. Studies in animals suggest that IL-1 may be particularly effective but its toxicity probably limits clinical use (Fibbe *et al.*, 1990). Preliminary data also suggest combined chemotherapy and GM- or G-CSF may allow efficient collection of large numbers of blood stem cells (Gianni *et al.*, 1989; Pettengell *et al.*, 1992).

How should blood stem cells be measured?

Eaves & Eaves (see Chapter 3) review the considerable difficulties in measuring hematopoietic stem cells in humans. Transplantation experiments in mice are more precise but not feasible in humans. Studies defining minimum numbers of cells for survival also cannot be performed in humans. Information is, however, available from studies which correlate hematopoietic reconstitution with numbers of blood stem cells and CFU-GM transplanted. Kessinger *et al.* (1989) reported reproducible hematopoietic reconstitution after blood stem cell infusions of more than 6×10^8 mononuclear cells/kg. When the blood stem cells are collected in steady state, this requires between six and ten aphereses. There appears to be no correlation between numbers of CFU-GM infused and hematopoietic reconstitution with steady state blood stem cells.

The CFU-GM assay is widely used to assess the quality and quantity of mobilized blood stem cell collections. Various authors recommend different minimum doses varying from 2×10^4 CFU-GM/kg in multiple myeloma (Fermand *et al.*, 1989) to 30×10^4 to 50×10^4 CFU-GM/kg in acute myeloid leukemia and lymphoma (To *et al.*, 1984). These CFU-GM doses correlate best with the time to neutrophil recovery. Correlations with platelet recovery are less impressive. Long-term hematopoietic reconstitution may be more related to survival of endogenous stem cells rather than the graft. Long-term reconstitution probably results from primitive stem cells not measured in the CFU-GM assay. Whether these come from the recipient, graft or both is uncertain.

Several new *in vitro* assays appear to correlate with stem cells responsible for longer term reconstitution. The competitive repopulating unit (CRU) assay in mice is an example. This assay is not feasible in humans, although gene marking studies may make such an approach possible in the future. The long-term culture initiating cell (LTC-IC) assay, where hematopoietic cells are cultured over fibroblast or bone marrow stromal layers for 5–8 weeks, with a CFU-GM assay performed on the supernatant cells after that period, correlates with the competitive repopulating unit assay and with long-term hematologic recovery in mice. The LTC-IC assay is used mostly to study normal hematopoiesis. There is a need to apply this approach to transplants.

An alternative approach is based on the pre CFU-GM or 'delta' assay.

The hematopoietic cell population of interest is cultured in medium with growth factors for 7 days and the cultured cells are then assayed for CFU-GM. The 'delta' or difference is the number of CFU-GM after 7 days compared with numbers of CFU-GM present at the beginning. The assay is thought to identify cells that are more primitive than CFU-GM. This approach also needs to be used to quantify blood stem cells and correlate them with transplant outcome.

Another approach is based on increasing knowledge of the phenotype of primitive hematopoietic cells. Developments in this area over the past 10 years are impressive. The most primitive hematopoietic stem cells appear to be $CD34^+$, $CD33^-$, $CD38^-$, DR^-, $Thy1^+$, rhodamine-low, and bear no markers of mature blood cells (lineage negative). Multiparameter cell sorting allows these subpopulations of cells to be quantified and their numbers correlated with hematopoietic reconstitution. Cells can also be sorted and studied in assays of LTC-IC and in the delta assay.

Collection of blood stem cells

There is vigorous debate about which machine and procedure is best to collect blood stem cells. These issues are discussed by To (see Chapter 6). Studies of collection efficiency have used many different approaches. Collection efficiency is usually in the range 60–70% irrespective of the machine or collection protocol. It is difficult to define the best method to collect blood stem cells when it is not known what cells are needed (as discussed). The best method of blood stem cell collection will have the fewest aphereses which collect the smallest numbers of cells needed for hematopoietic reconstitution. It is reasonable to assume that the fewer the cells collected, the less the likelihood of tumor contamination (as discussed by Sharp and Kessinger in Chapter 7). Also, collections and cryopreservations are time-consuming and expensive. Thus, it is important to attempt to collect blood stem cells when there are very high levels in the blood. Where studied carefully, with sequential daily assays, blood stem cell release is a dynamic process which is difficult to assess rapidly. The most commonly used measure, CFU-GM, requires 14 days of *in vitro* culture. Results are available only retrospectively. Indirect measures are based on correlations between blood stem cell release, white blood cell and platelet dynamics following chemotherapy. The pattern of hematologic recovery and blood stem cell release, however, varies considerably between patients and it is often difficult to be certain when it occurs. These problems may be less marked when blood stem cells are collected after use of hematopoietic growth factors. For example, G-CSF, 12 μg/kg per day, results in maximum progenitor cell release on days 5 to 7 (Sheridan *et al.*, 1992). An unproven alternative is to measure CD34$^+$ cells daily and begin apheresis when a threshold number of CD34$^+$ cells is reached. A rapid whole blood lysis method for CD34 measurement may help (Siena *et al.*, 1991).

Another issue related to blood stem cell collection is the volume of blood to be processed on each occasion. Obviously, the more blood is processed the more stem cells are collected. There is some evidence, however, to show that levels of mononuclear cells and CFU-GM fall during apheresis (Haylock *et al.*, 1992a). This requires further study.

Although the choice of blood cell separators may not be important, continuous flow devices are associated with less circulatory disturbance and more rapid processing. Blood stem cell collection is feasible using continuous flow devices in babies of less than 1 year of age (Emminger *et al.*, 1989; Takaue *et al.*, 1989). Those that are computer controlled are more likely to be successful with different operators. It seems reasonable to use a computer-controlled continuous flow cell separator which can process $\geqslant 10$ l in 2–3 h.

Blood stem cells are usually cryopreserved. This can cause problems when blood stem cell collections contain large numbers of granulocytes and monocytes, such as after hematopoietic growth factors. Some workers use density gradient separation before cryopreservation to remove contaminating cells. This results in less volume and a product more accurately assessed after thawing.

Hematopoietic reconstitution after blood stem cell transplants

There is no proof that autologous blood stem cells result in long-term hematopoietic reconstitution in humans. However, dogs transplanted with allogeneic unmobilized blood stem cells after high dose total body irradiation show complete donor reconstitution 10 years after a transplant (Carbonell *et al.*, 1984). In a mouse model using G-CSF-mobilized allogeneic blood stem cells, donor reconstitution is demonstrable beyond 1 year (Testa *et al.*, 1992). Preliminary data suggest that hematopoietic stem cells present in the blood may be more primitive than those in the bone marrow, on the basis of phenotype studies of CD34$^+$ subpopulations. Surprisingly, blood CD34$^+$ cells are typically rhodamine-low and show low levels of expression of mature lineage markers including CD33, whereas lower proportions of bone marrow CD34$^+$ cells are rhodamine-low and CD33 negative.

In humans the efficacy of mobilized transplants in producing rapid granulocyte recovery is well established. Several studies also demonstrate rapid platelet reconstitution but this is inconsistent and correlates less well with CFU-GM (To *et al.*, 1990b). These data suggest that there may be platelet stem cells which may not be comobilized with granulocyte stem cells. This deserves further study.

There are now many long-term human survivors of transplants. In Chapter 10, Hoyle and Goldman report 7–8-year survivors after transplants in chronic phase chronic myelogenous leukemia. Most subjects show at least some residual leukemia cells and it is uncertain whether the recovery resulted from the blood stem cell graft or endogenous hematopoiesis. The longest survival of transplants with a solid tumor is about 6 years (Korbling *et al.*, 1986). Long-term hematopoietic reconstitution after blood stem cell transplants is best studied after allogeneic transplants. The use of blood stem cells for allografts will almost certainly require T cell depletion because blood stem cell collections normally contain large numbers of T cells. There is a risk of increased graft-versus-host disease if too many, or of graft failure if too few, T cells are infused.

Stem cell selection

Selection of the cells that facilitate hematopoietic reconstitution after high dose treatment has a number of potential advantages (see Chapter 4). Stem cell selection may be an effective means of removing contaminating cancer cells. It may also provide cells useful for gene manipulation. As further information becomes available about subsets of hematopoietic stem cells responsible for the various stages of hematopoietic reconstitution, stem cell selection could enable one to tailor grafts to specific requirements. Selection may also yield cells ideally suited for *ex vivo* manipulation, such as expanding numbers of stem cells.

Current studies use enriched populations of $CD34^+$ cells. The techniques include magnetic beads and immunoabsorption on columns or rigid plastic. Purity lies between 60% and 95% and the yield is rarely better than 30–60% of $CD34^+$ cells processed. Hematopoietic reconstitution was demonstrated after transplants of $CD34^+$ bone marrow stem cells (Berenson *et al.*, 1991). Similar studies using blood stem cells are not yet reported. An additional benefit of selection is to reduce the number of cells for cryopreservation and the volume of dimethylsulfoxide (DMSO) given with the graft. Stem cell selection is an important area for future research.

Clinical results

Transplants have been widely used for only 6 to 8 years; nevertheless, hundreds of patients have been treated but unfortunately the design of trials limits the conclusions that can be drawn. In many cases, blood stem cells were combined with bone marrow. No randomized studies comparing autotransplants of blood stem cell versus bone marrow have been reported.

Conservative interpretation of currently available data suggests that blood stem cell autotransplants in acute myeloid leukemia produce similar leukemia-free survival to bone marrow autotransplants. Some studies show more rapid hematopoietic reconstitution with transplants but others do not. One nonrandomized study suggests an advantage for blood stem cell autotransplants in Hodgkin's disease and nonHodgkin's lymphoma. This requires confirmation. In multiple myeloma and breast cancer, blood stem cell autotransplants are largely used as an adjunct to bone marrow autotransplants. Studies of blood stem cells alone are progressing.

Cost

Blood stem cell autotransplants are often compared with bone marrow autotransplants. Three studies report significantly briefer hospitalizations with blood stem cell autotransplants, fewer days of fever, less antibiotic use and fewer transfusions (Elias *et al.*, 1992; Henon *et al.*, 1992; To *et al.*, 1992). These factors contribute to a substantial saving even if the cost of the mobilization procedures including cytokines, aphereses and multiple cryopreservation procedures is considered. Cost assessment was performed at the Dana-Farber Cancer Institute (Boston), the Royal Adelaide Hospital and the Hopital du Hasenrain, Mulhouse, France. In each case, the overall cost of transplants, including the multiple collection and cryopreservation procedures, was approximately one-half that of a bone marrow transplant. Many centres performing transplants still collect bone marrow, a substantial additional expense. This will become unnecessary as techniques for blood stem cell mobilization, collection and assessment improve.

Further directions

There are several important areas for future research. Little is understood about the mechanism of blood stem cell mobilization. Knowing how hematopoietic stem cells are released from the bone marrow into the blood may lead to better approaches. Preliminary data show important differences in the expression of adhesion molecules on bone marrow and blood stem cells. The best method of stem cell mobilization is controversial. G-CSF administration is simple, safe and predictable but combinations of growth factors may be better. The stem cell factor has been found to be very effective in primates. Combining G-CSF with chemotherapy may yield enough blood stem cells for reconstitution after high dose therapy with only a single apheresis.

The best collection technique and technology is also controversial. It requires improved techniques for assessment of hematopoietic reconstitution, numbers and 'quality' of stem cells, and level of tumor contamination. Dose intensification is widely studied in cancer therapy, but the best way to explore dose intensification is uncertain. *Ex vivo* stem cell manipulation may allow elimination of neutropenia and thrombocytopenia following high dose therapy (Haylock *et al.*, 1992b; Muench & Moore, 1992). This may permit novel approaches to high dose therapy. Repeated high dose therapy may be desirable, particularly in diseases like advanced breast cancer where conventional therapy is ineffective and in diseases which are more difficult to treat, such as advanced Hodgkin's disease and nonHodgkin's lymphoma. The repeated use of high dose therapy is likely to lead to unexpected and perhaps unpredictable nonhematopoietic toxicity (Pittman *et al.*, 1992) and it may be better to reduce the intensity of each high dose therapy. This concept could be tested using combined hematopoietic support including bone marrow, mobilized blood stem cells, *ex vivo* manipulation and hematopoietic growth factors.

Cost analysis remains an important issue and studies should include careful prospective collection of data. Quality of life may be assumed to be improved as a result of more rapid hematopoietic reconstitution but it is important that this be included in future studies.

Finally, when the technology of hematopoietic support for high dose therapy is optimized, it is important that large randomized studies compare this with standard treatment.

References

Berenson, R.J., Bensinger, W.I., Hill, R.S. *et al.* (1991). Engraftment after infusion of CD34$^+$ marrow cells in patients with breast cancer or neuroblastoma. *Blood*, **77**: 1717–22.

Brenner, M.K., Hill, D.R., Moen, R.C. *et al.* (1992). Applications of gene marking prior to autologous bone marrow transplantation. *J. Cell. Biochem.*, **16A**: 179 (abstract D029).

Bron, D., Philip, T., Guglielmi, C. *et al.* (1991). The Parma International Randomized Study in relapsed non Hodgkin lymphoma analysis on the first 153 pre-included patients. *Exp. Haematol.*, **19**: 546 (abstract 339).

Carbonell, F., Calvo, W., Fliedner, T.M. *et al.* (1984). Cytogenetic studies in dogs after total body irradiation and allogeneic transfusion with cryopreserved blood mononuclear cells: observations in long term chimeras. *Int. J. Cell Cloning*, **2**: 81–8.

Elias, A., Mazanet, R., Anderson, K. *et al.* (1992). GM-CSF mobilized peripheral blood stem cell autografts: the DFCI/BIH experience. *Int. J. Cell Cloning*, **10** (suppl. 1): 149–51.

Emminger, W., Emminger-Schmidmeier, W., Hocker, P., Hinterberger, W. & Gadner, H. (1989). Myeloid progenitor cells (CFU-GM) predict engraftment kinetics in autologous transplantation in children. *Bone Marrow Transplant.*, **4**: 415–20.

Fermand, J-P., Levy, Y., Gerota, J. *et al.* (1989). Treatment of aggressive multiple myeloma by high-dose chemotherapy and total body irradiation followed by blood stem cell autologous graft. *Blood*, **73**: 20–3.

Fibbe, W.E., Hamilton, M.S., Falkenburg, J.H.F. & Willemze, R. (1990). Sustained engraftment of mice transplanted with peripheral blood-derived interleukin-1 primed stem cells. *Exp. Hematol.*, **18**: 653 (abstract 398).

Gianni, A.M., Bregni, M., Siena, S. *et al.* (1991). Prospective randomized comparison of MACOP-B vs rhGM-CSF-supported high-dose sequential myeloablative chemo-radiotherapy in diffuse large cell lymphomas. *Proceedings of the American Society of Clinical Oncology.*, **10**: 274. (abstract 951).

Gianni, A.M., Siena, S., Bregni, M. *et al.* (1989). Granulocyte-macrophage colony-stimulating factor to harvest circulating haemopoietic stem cells for autotransplantation. *Lancet*, **2**: 580–5.

Gribben, J.G., Freedman, A.S., Neuberg, D. *et al.* (1991). Immunologic purging of marrow assessed by PCR before autologous bone marrow transplantation for B-cell lymphoma. *N. Engl. J. Med.*, **325**: 1525–33.

Gulati, S.C., Shank, B., Black, P. *et al.* (1988). Autologous bone marrow transplantation for patients with poor-prognosis lymphoma. *J. Clin. Oncol.*, **6**: 1303–13.

Haylock, D.N., Canty, A., Thorp, D., Dyson, P.G., Juttner, C.A. & To, L.B. (1992a). A discrepancy between the instantaneous and the overall collection efficiency of the Fenwal CS3000 for peripheral blood stem cell apheresis. *J. Clin. Apheresis*, **7**: 6–11.

Haylock, D.N., To, L.B., Dowse, T.L., Juttner, C.A. & Simmons, P.J. (1992b). Ex vivo expansion and maturation of peripheral blood CD34$^+$ cells into the myeloid lineage. *Blood*, **80**: 1405–12.

Henon, P.R., Liang, H., Beck-Wirth, G. *et al.* (1992). Comparison of hematopoietic and immune recovery after autologous bone marrow or blood stem cell transplants. *Bone Marrow Transplant.*, **9**: 285–91.

Horowitz, M.M., Gale, R.P., Sondel, P.M. *et al.* (1990). Graft-versus-leukaemia reactions after bone marrow transplantation. *Blood*, **75**: 555–62.

Hryniuk, W.M. (1988). The Importance of Dose Intensity in the Outcome of Chemotherapy in S. Hellman, V. De Vita, S. Rosenberg (eds): *Important Advances in Oncology*. Philadelphia, PA, Lippincott, 121–41.

Jagannath, S., Dicke, K.A., Armitage, J.O., Cabanillas, F.F., Horwitz, L.J., Vellekoop, L., Zander, A.R. & Spitzer, G. (1986). High-Dose Cyclophosphamide, Carmustine, and Etoposide and Autologous Bone Marrow Transplantation for Relapsed Hodgkin's Disease. *Annals of Internal Medicine*, **104**: 163–8.

Juttner, C.A., To, L.B., Haylock, D.N., Branford, A. & Kimber, R.J. (1985). Circulating autologous stem cells collected in very early remission from acute non-lymphoblastic leukaemia produce prompt but incomplete haemopoietic reconstitution after high dose melphalan or supralethal chemoradiotherapy. *Br. J. Haematol.*, **61**: 739–45.

Kessinger, A., Armitage, J.O., Smith, D.M., Landmark, J.D., Bierman, P.J. & Weisenburger, D.D. (1989). High dose therapy and autologous peripheral blood stem cell transplantation for patients with lymphoma. *Blood*, **74**: 1260–5.

Kolb, H.J., Mittermuller, J., Clemm, Ch. *et al.* (1990). Donor leukocyte transfusions for treatment of recurrent chronic myelogenous leukemia in marrow transplant patients. *Blood*, **76**: 2462–5.

Korbling, M., Dorken, B., Ho, A.D., Pezzutto, A., Hunstein, W. & Flidner, T.M. (1986). Autologous transplantation of blood-derived hemopoietic stem cells after myeloablative therapy in a patient with Burkitt's lymphoma. *Blood*, **67**: 529–32.

Muench, M.M. & Moore, M.A.S. (1992). Accelerated recovery of peripheral blood cell counts in mice transplanted with in vitro cytokine-expanded hematopoietic progenitors. *Exp. Hematol.*, **20**: 611–18.

Pettengell, R., Demuynck, H., Testa, N.G. & Dexter, T.M. (1992). The engraftment capacity of peripheral blood progenitor cells mobilized with chemotherapy G-CSF. *Int. J. Cell Cloning*, **10** (suppl. 1): 59–61.

Pittman, K.B., To, L.B., Bayly, J.L. *et al.* (1992). Non-haematological toxicity limiting the application of sequential high dose chemotherapy in patients with advanced breast cancer. *Bone Marrow Transplant.*, **10**: 535–40.

Reiffers, J., Bernard, P., David, B. *et al.* (1986). Successful autologous transplantation with peripheral blood hemopoietic cells in a patient with acute leukaemia. *Exp. Hematol.*, **14**: 312–15.

Sheridan, W.P., Begley, C.G., Juttner, C.A. *et al.* (1992). Effect of peripheral-blood progenitor cells mobilized by Filgrastim (G-CSF) on platelet recovery after high dose chemotherapy. *Lancet*, **339**: 640–4.

Siena, S., Bregni, M., Brando, B. *et al.* (1991). Flow cytometry for clinical estimation of circulating hematopoietic progenitors for autologous transplantation in cancer patients. *Blood*, **77**: 400–9.

Socinski, M.A., Cannistra, S.A., Elias, A., Antman, K.H., Schnipper, L. & Griffin, J.D. (1988). Granulocyte-macrophage colony-stimulating factor expands the circulating haemopoietic progenitor cell compartment in man. *Lancet*, **1**: 1194–8.

Takaue, Y., Watanabe, T., Kawano, Y. *et al.* (1989). Isolation and storage of peripheral blood hematopoietic stem cells for autotransplantation into children with cancer. *Blood*, **74**: 1245–51.

Testa, N.G., Molineu, G., Hampson, I.N., Lord, B.I. & Dexter, T.M. (1992). Comparative assessment and analysis of peripheral blood and bone marrow stem cells. *Int. J. Cell Cloning*, **10** (suppl. 1): 30–4.

To, L.B., Haylock, D.N., Dyson, P.G., Thorp, D., Roberts, M. & Juttner, C.A. (1990a). An unusual pattern of haemopoietic reconstitution in patients with acute myeloid leukaemia transplanted with autologous recovery phase peripheral blood. *Bone Marrow Transplant.*, **6**: 109–14.

To, L.B., Haylock, D.N., Kimber, R.J. & Juttner, C.A. (1984). High levels of circulating haemopoietic stem cells in very early remission from acute non-lymphoblastic leukaemia and their collection and cryopreservation. *Br. J. Haematol.*, **58**: 399–410.

To, L.B., Juttner, C.A., Stomski, F., Vadas, M.A. & Kimber, R.J. (1987). Immune reconstitution following peripheral blood stem cell autografting. *Bone Marrow Transplant.*, **2**: 111–12 (letter).

To, L.B., Roberts, M.M., Haylock, D.N. *et al.* (1992). Comparison of haematology recovery times and supportive care requirements of autologous recovery phase peripheral blood stem cell transplants, autologous bone marrow transplants and allogeneic bone marrow transplants. *Bone Marrow Transplant.*, **9**: 277–84.

To, L.B., Sheppard, K.M., Haylock, D.N. *et al.* (1990b). Single high doses of cyclophosphamide enable the collection of high numbers of haemopoietic stem cells from the peripheral blood. *Exp. Hematol.*, **18**: 442–7.

Index

181